EVERYONE
HATES
THE
DENTIST

EVERYONE
HATES
THE
DENTIST

TOM DISTEFANO DMD

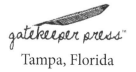
gatekeeper press™
Tampa, Florida

Everyone Hates The Dentist

Published by Gatekeeper Press
7853 Gunn Hwy., Suite 209
Tampa, FL 33626
www.GatekeeperPress.com

Library of Congress Control Number: 2024935038

ISBN (paperback): 9781662950933
eISBN: 9781662950940

Acknowledgements

I WOULD LIKE to thank many people for the contributions made by them in the creation of this book.

First and foremost, I would like to thank my parents, Lou and Louise, for raising me, inspiring me to visualize my goals, and providing me with the resources, opportunity, and education needed to accomplish them.

I would also like to thank all of the employees and associates that helped me provide the dentistry about which I've written.

I would also be remiss if I did not recognize the patients that placed their trust in me and shared their lives with me.

Finally, I would like to thank Donna Sobol for having the interest and faith in my story and pushing me to make this book actually happen rather than end up on the junk pile of unfinished good ideas.

Table of Contents

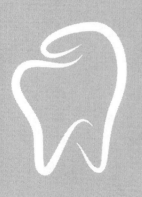

PART ONE

THE PEOPLE

Why We Are the Way We Are

WE AS DENTISTS are a unique group. We work in an environment made stressful by complicated interpersonal interactions and the fears of pain and cost. Perhaps not the sort of life-threatening, stressful environment that soldiers, policemen, and firefighters deal with but a more insidious, constant, multifaceted version of stress. Some people fear us and not enough appreciate us. All most people want is to have as little to do with us as possible. They want to get away from us as quickly as they can. A visit with us has become synonymous with a torture session or some other unpleasantry in common culture. This can make us appear and feel somewhat different from other people. We are also simultaneously tasked with the responsibilities of running a business and working effectively within the myriad interpersonal relationships in our office.

For better or worse, this pressure cooker eventually forges us into someone different from who we were when we started practicing. That evolution may be one of softening, and developing a higher level of consciousness, or it may go the other way, souring us to develop a bitter, self-centered, and petty outlook. I've seen it go both ways. It depends on how you handle what life throws you and probably starts with who you are inherently. The raw materials matter. I believe it takes a bit of an OCD, high-strung, perfectionist sort of person to be drawn to this profession in the first place. During the process of applying to dental school, the interviewers asked questions to determine just how meticulous you were. Obviously, your grades needed to be high enough to be accepted into these very competitive positions. They were looking for more than just grades, though. That could be found on the transcripts and resumes; they didn't need an interview for that. Maybe they were looking for some hint of the traits of intensity and focus that this profession demands. Most people don't get grades this high by relaxing and coasting through their obligations and responsibilities. I'm not necessarily saying that preparing to try to get accepted into dental school makes you crazy, but I think those that do walk that path are a bit more inherently serious and intense. Think of Hermey from *Rudolph the Red-Nosed Reindeer*. Nice enough, but a little off, no? Definitely not the funniest elf in Santa's workshop. I remember those first days of dental school, getting to know many of my classmates and seeing the sort of people they were. Most of them came in pretty high-strung, and there were more than just a few Hermeys in that group.

As the weeks, months, and years in school went on, the further "development" occurred. We were constantly taught that nothing we did was good enough. We were required to always make it a little (or a lot) better. Ostensibly, this was done to further hone our skills and teach us to be more discerning and to always strive to achieve something closer to perfection in a tiny imperfect region of a very imperfect world.

But the methodology of this indoctrination was not always kind. The requirements were often very stringent and inflexible. Worse yet, the personal judgments by those holding the reins to our progress were often very subjective. Interactions with some instructors could vary from favoritism to barely hidden unwarranted hostility. There was nepotism, sexism, tribalism, and just plain meanness. The anxiety builds as you start to feel like maybe you don't belong there. You begin to wonder if all those years of trying to get in were wasted. You worry about how ashamed you'll be if you fail. You start to feel that if you fail as a dentist, the only job you will be qualified for with your biology degree is to clean out rat cages. The concept of educating dental students is often consciously or unconsciously replaced with hazing them. There is a compulsion on the part of some instructors that makes them feel like it's their duty to battle-harden or weed out the weak, like some sort of drill sergeant or fraternity hazing officer. We were asked things like "Don't you have a relative that can get you into a different career?" and were looked at with a bewildered expression that seemed to scream "How the hell did they let you in here?" If you didn't come in with an inferiority complex, you could certainly develop one.

And then you start to get a taste of what it means to be a dentist. How it feels to stick people with sharp instruments. What it's like to cut them and watch them bleed. What goes through your head during an impression as you try to get them to hold on and fight the gag reflex long enough for it to be accurate while hoping they don't throw up on you. You're introduced to the wonderful world of trying to focus intently on the tooth you're drilling while simultaneously spending more of your focus on keeping the tongue and cheek from wandering onto the cutting edge of the drill. All the while, you're aware that sometimes the patient erupts like a jack-in-the-box, twitching, jumping, and maybe even grabbing your hand.

You learn to use nuances in language, choosing words like "slight discomfort" rather than "pain" or "hurt." You learn to add the word "much" when forced to say "discomfort" so as to minimize the threat. But to some extent, you're bluffing. Like Forrest Gump's box of chocolates, you're never quite sure what you're going to get. You don't really know whether they will actually feel the injection, how they will perceive it, or best of all, whether it will even work.

The first few extractions that you and your classmates perform are always eye-openers. You've already been taught the hows and whys of the technique, but until you actually do one or at least see it being done in person, you never really know how it's going to hit you. The sight of blood and the ickiness of the feeling can have unexpected effects on you. I suppose human dissection on cadavers in freshman-year gross anatomy prepares you a bit for that, but corpses don't bleed and you don't have to worry about hurting or killing them. There's always a bit of trepidation and some degree of nausea and faintness, but the full-out fainters in your group of novice tooth pullers are the best! You ridicule your fainting comrades mercilessly, never admitting that you weren't that far off. Eventually, it seems that everyone kind of gets past that, and they let you loose on the general public on a mission to remove all the troubled, hopeless teeth of this world (or at least as many as it takes to complete your requirements). You go through the motions you were taught, using instruments to gently expand the socket and loosen the ligaments and the tooth to the point that it can delicately be removed from the jaw, just like in the video. But sometimes it doesn't work that way. You can't see. You can't get the instrument in at the angle you would like to. You're not even sure that you're using the right instrument, and in time, there's a pile of instruments on the table that you've unsuccessfully tried. Yet the tooth still refuses to budge. And then comes the dreaded noise, CRACK!!! The root breaks. You hear it break, but you feel it even more. You feel it from your fingers through your hand and wrist and all the way to your elbow. The tooth breaks deep, where you can't even see it, let alone get to it and remove it. A flood of emotions and thoughts rush through your mind at this point, not the least of which is regret for choosing this miserable career path. But at this point, you reach deep inside yourself and do what you gotta do to get yourself out of this dilemma. It may involve a deeper surgical access to go get it or the diligent, patient use of root tip picks or even a strategic retreat, shamefully handing it over to the oral surgery instructor overseeing you. He'll probably make you try the first two options first, but he knows full well ahead of time whether you actually have a chance of succeeding or whether you'll spend the next twenty minutes needlessly torturing and maiming the poor bastard in your chair while you learn your lesson. Fun stuff.

You eventually emerge from the meat grinder of dental school and venture out into the world as a dentist. You feel like you've paid your dues and eagerly look forward to your wealthy cruise down easy street. Little do you know that this is when playtime ends and the real world starts.

First of all, you're faced with a very sudden shift in your identity or at least the one you are supposed to present. You are suddenly not that twenty-two-year-old, fun-loving kid you used to be. You might be able to relate with him for a little while despite keeping him bottled up inside, but eventually he'll wither and die, stifled under the doctor costume and the responsibilities that come with it. You are a now a doctor with a license to stab, cut, drill, and charge people as you see fit. You need to be able to inspire people with your knowledge and experience (of which you have precious little at this point). So you dress properly, speak properly, and do your best. It can be difficult at first trying to carry yourself with an identity you're not used to and don't really believe in yet. You talk the talk as convincingly as you can. The one thing that keeps you from being even more unsure of yourself is that, as a young person, you don't even know what you don't know. There are so many mistakes you haven't made yet and so many troublesome people to meet and sticky situations yet to get into. Your clueless bravado usually works to some extent, but it certainly has its limitations.

What I came to discover was that the sweet spot of impressive personal presentation is different for a young dentist rather than for an older dentist. When you're young, if you don't show quite enough confidence, you will be viewed as unsure and inexperienced. Too much confidence and you will seem brash and cocky. The younger you are, the narrower the safe zone between these danger zones is. As a result, you focus on trying to find a way to present yourself as neither of those. For the older dentist, the out of bounds seem to be arrogance versus appearing out of touch, outdated, or beyond your prime. But the size of the golden power zone between those negative projected perceptions seems to vary over time. Since it is very narrow in the beginning of your career when you are young, the twenty-six-year-old kid is at a disadvantage here. All the older dentist has to do is display his knowledge in a polite and caring way and not be too obnoxious about it. And he also has the advantage that he has been playing the part a lot longer and probably knows a little more about his audience. Speaking of his audience, he has already treated most of his patients for a long time and barely has to prove himself. They will almost always give him the benefit of the doubt.

We begin our careers ambitious and armed with a diploma and a goal of succeeding as a dentist. We are anxiously hoping to prove those years and dollars of schooling were worth it all. We go to work and begin to ply our new trade as best we can. The faculty's primary responsibility had been to teach us all the technical and didactic aspects of dentistry. Unfortunately, practice management and the subtle nuances of the unique interpersonal interactions in dentistry were not in the syllabus of covered subjects. You might have learned some of that in the conversations you may have had with some of the more amicable and chatty instructors. There was even more to be learned by simply watching some of your instructors as they interacted with patients. If you engaged these instructors, you just might have learned something valuable. Sometimes it was a technical tip. Other times, it was patient management advice or even just plain old charm and showmanship. I remember one situation in particular where I was adjusting a denture that a patient was complaining irrationally about. The instructor came over and asked her what was wrong. She recited her litany of complaints in a much more respectful tone to him. He nodded understandingly and told her we would fix it in the lab. As he and I entered the lab, he told me that it was a "one butt adjustment." He tossed the denture on the lab bench, went out the back door, smoked one butt, and then came back in, grabbed the denture with his bare nicotine-stained fingers and gave it to the patient, who was very satisfied with what this wonderfully experienced dentist had done for her. Experiences like this with these seasoned instructors sometimes showed you what to do. Other times, they showed you what not to do. It's up to you to figure it out. Much of our education and development before and after graduation involved getting into situations, working as hard as we could to find our way out of them, and learning on the fly, oblivious to the next pitfall that may lie ahead.

I realize that the timeline in this chapter seems to bounce around a bit between pre- and post-graduation, and I apologize for the confusion it may cause. The truth is that this chapter speaks about education and development, and they have no finite limits. We are constantly learning and changing. Certain topics drift in and out of our focus, but we are never truly completely knowledgeable about any of them, regardless of age or student status.

As time goes on, you come to see what a jack-of-all-trades you must be in order to succeed as a dentist. First and foremost, you need to be proficient in the technical aspects of dentistry. For that, you need to be an engineer, a chemist, and a sculptor. You need to possess the heart and mind of an artist to be able to envision beauty and his hands and perseverance to create it. You also need to be an engineer, a biologist, an electrician, and a builder in order to understand and physically make it all work. The interpersonal aspects of what we do require you to be a counselor, a life coach, a teacher, a psychologist, an accountant, and a financial advisor to name but a few. The ability to wear many hats and perform costume changes as you move repeatedly from one task and patient to the next is not easy but can endear you to your patients and employees. The ability to read the moods and attitudes from one person to the next and then match those traits is called mirroring and is essential and incredibly powerful.

Let me tell you a few stories about some of the early patient experiences that, for better or worse, helped to mold me into the dentist I am today.

The Crazies

IT WAS MY first year in the very small practice that I had bought. It was at the end of the day, at about 6 p.m., and everyone in the rest of the building had gone home. The hallways were quiet and a little dark. My staff members (both of them) had gone home, and I was doing paperwork. I had plans to go to my mom's for dinner.

The door to my office opened, and in walked a man who could best be described as Uncle Fester from *The Addams Family*, except that this guy looked crazier. He asked if he could get his teeth cleaned. I explained that the office was closed for the day, but I would be glad to schedule him an appointment. He again asked if he could get his teeth cleaned that night. I relented, figuring I could get it done in a little while, and agreed to clean his teeth immediately. After all, I was trying to build a practice and was willing to do whatever it took in order to do so. He filled out the forms, and I brought him in. As I did his exam, I noticed two things. One, his teeth had minimal accumulation of plaque. Two, he was even more bizarre than I first thought. The phone rang. It was my mom, asking where I was. I told her I'd be a little late and why. I noticed on the "new patient" form that this guy lived on the same street as a friend of hers, and I told her so. I went back into the treatment room and finished his cleaning. He asked when he could get them cleaned again. I told him six months. He asked if he could get them cleaned in one month and I told him no, that he barely needed them cleaned today.

He told me his bite was off and asked if I could adjust it. I asked where. He pointed to one tooth. I adjusted it. He pointed to another. And another. I barely adjusted those, and he asked when he could get his teeth cleaned again. I, yet again, told him six months. He inquired as to whether he could come back in only one month for another cleaning. I told him that would be unnecessary. He asked again about his bite. I told him I already fixed it. We were caught in a loop. He then informed me that his teeth were sensitive. I asked which teeth. He pointed to one, and I placed desensitizing gel on it. Then he pointed to another and another. Soon I was applying desensitizing gel to all of his teeth. Predictably, at this point, he asked me when he could get his teeth cleaned again.

At that point, the phone rang again. It was my mom. She had checked with the friend who lived on the same street and told me, "Get him out of there! He just got released from a mental institution, where he was sent because he tried to kill his parents and set their house on fire."

I briefly contemplated simply leaving the office and calling the police, but then I settled on a better idea. I took one of my business cards and wrote the name and number of a nearby dentist who had given me a hard time when he was an instructor at my dental school and I was a student. I went back into the room, gave him the card, and explained to him that I was just on the phone with the best dentist I knew, who was probably the only dentist in the area who could handle his unique set of needs. I purposely wrote the dentist's name and number on my card and instructed him to present the card and be sure to tell that dentist that I had sent him.

During that first year that I was practicing, I was splitting my time between my office and the office of an older dentist's. One day, when we were both working on different patients in adjacent rooms, I could hear what was going on in his room. His patient was becoming increasingly and irrationally agitated, loudly asking, "What is that!!?? What are you doing???"

He calmly reassured her that it was only a piece of cotton and a mirror. He told her that he was only taking a look. He steered the appointment to a close, and the assistant escorted her to the front of the office.

A moment later, she ran back into the operatory screaming, "You think I don't know you called the f*****g cops???" Without a moment's hesitation, he nonchalantly lifted the phone off the receiver on the wall and spoke calmly into the dial tone and said, "It's ok, she's gone." It satisfied her, and she simply walked out of the office, never to return.

Getting the crazies out of the office is the primary objective at that point. Say whatever you have to say, do whatever you have to do in order to get them moving toward the door.

An ounce of prevention is worth a pound of cure. We are certainly not trained for these sorts of situations, but in the emotionally supercharged world of dentistry, we are sometimes presented with them. There are many factors to assess when trying to deal with them. First of all, being able to see them coming a little earlier and, therefore, avoid them is certainly very helpful. Look in their eyes when they speak, and learn to notice, read, and understand many of the facial expressions that they may show you. Reviewing the medications that a new patient is taking is essential. It will very often be your first clue as to what you may be dealing with. Paying extraordinary attention to every detail when you first speak to a patient is also very important. Reading between the lines regarding not only the words that they use but also figuring out why they choose them is a bit of a learned skill. If something seems off or doesn't add up, chase it down a bit, and learn more about it. It is much better to learn it during the consultation than midway through a dental procedure.

The Nasties

ANOTHER TIME in that office, I was scheduled to do a crown insert on a very grouchy businessman. He had taken off time from work and was already seated when I got to the office. The assistants were panicking because his crown had not come back from the lab (most likely because it had not been sent there on time). I soon joined them in their panic. What were we to do? The older dentist came in and inquired as to what the problem was. We explained, and he simply asked for a piece of warm wax. We tried to explain again that the crown was not there. He calmly waved us off and walked into the operatory, and before the patient could utter a word, he stuck the wax into the patient's mouth and told him to bite. While the patient's mouth was stuffed with wax, he explained that he was not satisfied with the crown that the lab had sent and that he wanted to confirm the bite registration, probably adding something like "Nothing but the best for you, Bill." He told him he would see him in a week. He told him to open, and he removed the wax and quickly walked out of the operatory. The quick thinking and the stage presence was very impressive. But the pièce de résistance was the way he casually tossed the wax "prop" into the trash just outside the patient's field of view, like an actor once he was behind the curtain.

While I cannot necessarily publicly extol dishonesty, there are times where the narrative needs to be shifted in the name of pragmatism. Should the irritability of a patient coupled with a delay from the lab result in the loss of a patient from the practice and the subsequent diminishment of the reputation of the practice? I suppose that is morally debatable. But this is a book about practice management and interesting anecdotes, not morality and ethics, so it stays.

Billy B. was the worst, most miserable patient of my career. I should have seen it from a mile away, but I was young, naïve, and stupid. The stink of negativity hovered around him like a pungent cloud, but I had not yet learned to recognize that particular stench nor the magnitude of misery it foretold.

The first time he came in, he was carrying a bag of three sets of dentures and he launched into a diatribe about how terrible the dentures and the dentists who had made them were. Thinking that I could do a better job than the others was my commission of the crime of hubris. Time would prove that ignorance of the law was no defense, and I was to be appropriately punished. Over the multiple appointments involved in the fabrication of the dentures, he made the time he spent with me a living hell. Procedurally, he was a nightmare. He gagged, grabbed my hand, and pulled it from his mouth in the middle of impressions. He fought me as I tried to take a bite registration, never closing the same way twice but always clamping down as hard as he could and smashing the wax rims. At the wax set up visit, I turned my back on him for a moment only to turn around and find him pulling the denture teeth out of the wax and throwing them onto the table.

These procedural disasters paled in comparison to the emotional misery he spewed nonstop. He complained about the weather. He complained about his job. He complained about his ex-wife. He complained about the government, his boss, and the stairs in the office. This constant torrent of negativity cascaded endlessly out of his miserable toothless mouth, like the discharge from a filthy polluted sewer pipe. It got to the point that if I saw his name on the schedule for the next day, that day was already ruined, regardless of whom else might be there.

Somehow, miraculously, I finished the dentures without killing him or myself. Two days later, he barged into the waiting room demanding to see me. Thankfully, there were no other patients in the office. I asked him what the problem was, and he complained that these dentures were just as bad as all the others and that he wasn't paying for them. I quietly asked him to hand me the dentures and confirmed that he had no intention of paying. He confirmed.

I remember how the plastic dentures looked as they flew across the room and shattered as they hit the old, plaster walls. I don't remember how it sounded, but that's probably because I was screaming at him to get the hell out of my office.

There are so many lessons to be learned from this one. First and foremost, it is crucial to spot the troublemakers before they infect your life. This can sometimes be tricky because they're usually on their best behavior in the beginning. But this one was miserable from the get-go, and I got what I deserved for missing it. The audacity of thinking I could do better before knowing what I was getting into was another lesson learned. Sun Tzu said that you must count before you calculate, calculate before you plan, and plan before you execute. It is amazing to me how often we all fail to properly follow this most simple protocol in so many varied aspects of our lives.

Misery Loves Company

I AM NOT sure whether I believe in the old saying that "misery loves company." Misery certainly can spread misery, and miserable people often intentionally or unintentionally create misery in the people around them. But I don't think misery actually loves company. Misery loves nothing. Misery is darkness and loneliness. It is shameful, and it craves and creates its own solitude and isolation. It is, by definition, the antithesis of love and enjoyment. No three words are less suited to inhabit the same sentence than misery, love, and company.

Given its toxicity and the flood of harmful neurotransmitters it initiates into your body, one should learn to spot misery and do all you can to avoid it. See it as the scourge that it is. Recognize it in all its forms. Be unavailable to it. Discourage it. Belittle and ridicule it. Banish it from your practice and your life whenever possible.

Alien Root Canals

I ONCE HAD a new patient that we took a full set of X-rays on during her first visit. It was immediately evident that, among other previous dental work, she had had three root canals done. When I mentioned that to her, she sternly corrected me, saying, "No, I've only had two." I showed her the X-rays and pointed to all of them, counting "one, two, and three." She adamantly responded, "I would have known if I had a third root canal!"

At this point, I had several options as to how to proceed. I could continue to argue with her and try to educate her as to how root canals and radiology worked. But after she showed me how closed-minded, stubborn, and belligerent she was during the first two exchanges, I had very little faith or interest in that path. My second choice would be to swallow my dignity and agree to the idiotic opinion that there were only two root canals in that set of X-rays.

Neither of those options appealed to me, and I was starting to recognize our friend from the last section: misery. So I chose option three. I gave it one last shot to see if in fact that was what I was dealing with. I asked her if she had ever been outside at night and saw a bright light in the sky. She reluctantly and unhappily said, "I guess so." I nodded thoughtfully and said, "Ah, I see. That must have been the night the aliens beamed you up to their ship and did the third root canal. It's really quite good by their standards."

She was not amused. She did not return to the office. Good riddance. Better to be rid of such a negative person nice and early before she had a chance to further pollute my life by arguing and challenging everything I said or did with no regard for reason.

It is not that I cannot tolerate someone who disagrees with me. In fact, I very often welcome a dissenting rational opinion. We can all certainly learn from knowledgeable, intelligent people with experiences and opinions other than our own. What can you possibly learn from someone who already thinks exactly as you do? But the new point of view must be rational and make logical sense on some level in order to earn my respect and be worthy of my contemplation and conversation. In the end, we do owe them a complete and thorough explanation of how we intend to treat them and our best efforts in the delivery of care but not a lot more.

The Harmless

THEY'RE NOT all bad. In fact, far from it. You really do meet so many interesting people in this business and hear some funny and interesting things. If time permits, it can be pretty entertaining to listen a bit. With open ears and an open mind, you can learn a lot about people from these encounters.

I once had an elderly patient in the chair, and I was reviewing her "new patient" form with her. She had left the date of birth blank. When I asked her what her date of birth was, she got up from the chair, stepped into the storage closet, and gestured for me to follow her in there. I was puzzled by the bizarre request but complied just to be polite. I was reasonably sure I wasn't in danger as she didn't appear to be armed, and I was pretty sure I could beat her in a fight. Once we were both in there, she whispered that she was seventy-four years old, but she had told her gentleman friend that she was only sixty-nine. He was in the waiting room and had been there while she was filling the form out. She didn't want him to hear her tell me that she was seventy-four. To me, a twenty-six-year-old guy, it didn't seem like such a big deal. But to her, it meant a lot. I'm sure that, in her mind, the strength of her relationship rested on it. The stakes couldn't have been higher for her, and it wasn't important to me, so we noted her date of birth elsewhere and promised to keep her secret. Why not? The point is, sometimes people have reasons that are very important to them when they do or say things that might seem quite bizarre or meaningless to the rest of us. It is usually best to give them the benefit of the doubt and try to communicate and let them express themselves en route to a better understanding and stronger relationship.

The world of dentistry can be filled with amusing accidental double entendre phrases. At least, I think they were accidental. I usually just let them pass so as to not embarrass the person who said it. In the name of good taste, I won't quote them here. Let your imagination run wild and know that the actual utterances were probably a little worse.

I've also expanded my vocabulary as a result of interacting with patients. For example, I learned what "He's going away" meant when they cleared my schedule for two days so that I could do a month's worth of work on a certain somewhat dangerous-looking patient, who I was told was "going away." I asked why such a hurry when was he coming back? The patient laughed and said, "The judge said ten years with good behavior."

And then there is the mental multitasking. I once had a patient stare into my eyes constantly while I worked. It was very unnerving. Turns out, she was simply looking at the reflection in my glasses to watch what was going on in her mouth. But she was gorgeous, so that made it a bit more distracting. But not nearly as unnerving as it got when she told me she practiced witchcraft. Talk about multiple challenges to concentration!

Watch Your Mouth

WHEN INTERACTING with people on a personal basis, especially within the constraints of a long-term professional relationship, it's important to think before you speak. It's amazing how stupid and insensitive some of the things that can fall out of your mouth can be if you're not careful.

I once had an elderly couple that had been coming to the practice since before I bought it. The husband became very ill and was hospitalized. I was in the process of making a set of dentures for the wife. Over the course of several weeks, she would come to her appointment with me in the morning and then go visit him at the hospital in the afternoon. This was the pattern right up until the day that I gave her the finished dentures. For some reason, I checked the obituaries a day or two after that last visit. Sure enough, the husband was listed among the recently deceased. He had passed away. A few months later when his son was in, I offered my condolences. He thanked me and said, "Yeah, Mom too." I was flabbergasted and said, "No! When?" He told me the date. Time had passed, and I could not believe she had been gone several months. It felt like she had just been in the office receiving the dentures. Turned out, she had died of a broken heart just a few days after her husband did. Any sane, compassionate individual would have extended the condolences to include the mom and left it at that. But not this idiot. I argued with this man that he must be mistaken about the date of his mother's death, even going so far as to pull her chart to try to prove that she had just been in. To this day, I can still remember the taste of my foot in my mouth.

The point of the story is that, especially in such close quarters and regarding such personal matters, one should always pause and think before speaking.

Another patient that I remember came in one day and was unusually quiet. Usually cheerful and bubbly, something was missing. I generally find myself pretty aware of the mood of people around me. Two sentences in, I could tell something was a little off. Many times, I will tell a joke or a story or try to come up with something charming to say in order to break the ice and lighten the mood in the room. But I had a feeling this was different, and a little voice in my head told me to back off and tread lightly. After a bit, I very quietly and compassionately asked if she was ok. She began to sob and told me that her husband had died the day before. Thank God for that little voice and my developing sense to heed it.

Much later in life, I had a patient who needed several dental procedures. I explained them to her, and she seemed very interested in getting them done. But she would cancel her appointments after getting one or two things done and disappear for several months before reappearing and repeating the cycle. As disappointing as it was to not be able to provide her with the care that she needed and wanted, we never gave her a hard time for her disappearances. We simply welcomed her back like Little Bo Peep's sheep or the Prodigal Son in the Bible. Maybe it was her likeable demeanor, maybe it was a desire to help her at all costs, or maybe I had just gotten a lot better at listening to that soft little cautious voice in my head. As it turned out, we later found out that she had a child with a serious medical condition that demanded 150 percent of her time and effort when it flared up. Beyond listening to the little voice, there is a lot to be said for developing a sense of tolerance and patience when dealing with people and the complex lives they may lead.

That sense of tolerance and patience is not very complicated. It simply involves paying attention to the other person and having some sense of humanity. If a person does not seem to want to engage in conversation or seems a little sad or off after an attempt or two to connect, then by all means, let it go! You have no idea what is going on in someone else's life. Sometimes they are dealing with something very difficult for them, and sometimes they just don't feel like talking. You should generally try to engage but also be very aware of when it's time to disengage. Unless you're invited in, butt out! It's none of your business. Discretion and compassion can never be faulted and will always gain the hearts and minds of others.

Oldies but Goodies

THE DENTIST whose practice I bought was in his early seventies. His name was William Brucker, and he was the consummate gentleman. Respected and loved in the community, he was a learned and very intelligent man. There was an innate kindness and geniality to him. Quick-witted, poetic, and affable, he loved his patients, the arts, and humanity in general. Several conversations with him helped to further shape my attitude toward my patients. These conversations were thinly veiled interrogations of me as a potential buyer and steward of his practice and showed a deep concern for his patients. These were people he had cared for for nearly fifty years. He needed to know that they would continue to be treated with the same level of consideration and dignity that they had always enjoyed under his tenure. Experiencing that concerned vetting process reinforced in me a sense of responsibility that I am proud to say I still carry and will very likely instill in my successor.

Being fortunate enough to have all four of my grandparents in my life until I was nearly thirty may have led to some of my understanding, appreciation, and opinions toward the elderly. My father's father died when I was twenty-five and he ninety-three. The other three lived at least ten more years until I was in my late thirties and they in their late eighties. They all lived nearby, and I was close with all of them. Subsequently, I connected very naturally with many of the elderly patients in the practice that I bought. Most of these older people had a quiet dignity about them, rarely complaining and virtually never appearing afraid of their impending fate. Some even joked about it, telling me that they read the obituaries at the beginning of every day, and as long as they didn't see their own names, it was going to be a good day. Others chuckled as they mentioned being so old that they didn't buy green bananas anymore.

But the golden years are not always golden. There was one gentleman that comes to mind named Joseph. He was in his late eighties and came in one day very depressed. When I asked him if he was ok, he told me that he was very lonely. His wife had died, his friends had died, and he was living in his daughter's house with a son-in-law that he was sure resented him being there. He asked how my grandmother was. She had just passed away very suddenly and comfortably at the age of eighty-seven after living an incredibly healthy life, and I told him so. Joseph expressed his condolences but also said that to live such a long, healthy life and pass quickly without suffering was a very good deal. He said it was a deal he would gladly take. A few months later, his daughter came in, and I asked her how her dad was, telling her how depressed he had been when I last saw him. She told me that he had died very suddenly of a massive stroke several months earlier. I expressed my condolences and shut my mouth. I did, however, wonder if I had given him the idea about that deal. I certainly made no mention of that part of our conversation. I was learning.

Many of the interactions and relationships that I had with some of the older patients were some of the most rewarding moments of my career and life. All many of these people want is to be paid attention to, be told that they matter, and be listened to. Much of it is unspoken.

The appreciation that comes from providing the consideration that they crave is unmistakable. Often, I have found a strength and a sense of class from the people of this "greatest generation."

I once had a new patient in his eighties call for an appointment to get a tooth pulled. I told him I would be glad to take a look. He brusquely replied that "You can look all you want, but I'm coming to get the tooth pulled!" Before he arrived, I called the oral surgeon next door and confirmed that he would be available to extract the tooth if needed. The patient showed up and marched into my treatment room. I looked at the tooth, and it did indeed require extraction. He asked if I would pull the tooth. I replied "no" and paused for effect. His face flashed with rage, and I completed my sentence, telling him that I had already arranged for the oral surgeon to take care of him and they were standing by, waiting for him. The part that I just left out was that, although he was in his eighties and about five foot seven and maybe one hundred thirty-five pounds, he stood ramrod straight, and there was not a hint of a wrinkle in his perfectly ironed clothes. Turned out, he had been a decorated fighter pilot in World War II. An Ace, in fact. A unique and impressive individual indeed.

Mr. and Mrs. M were longtime and beloved patients. A kinder, more considerate, happier couple never lived. One very hot summer day, when her denture was returned from the lab, rather than making them drive twenty miles to my office to get it, I offered to deliver it to them, as I had a few errands to run in that direction. Well, the delivery turned into a tour of the house and garden and a glass of wine. And of course, a nice glass of wine demands a big plate of spaghetti. I never got to those other errands. Oh well.

Angelo was another good one. He came in on a Monday morning with several badly broken front teeth. His lip had been lacerated and had already scabbed over. I asked what had happened, and he angrily said that he stupidly tripped on a curb and fell face-first. Noting the degree of scabbing, I asked him when it had happened. He replied that it was Friday, three days earlier. I scolded him for not calling me immediately. He waved me off and simply said, "Nah, it was the weekend, didn't want to bother you."

Maria was an elderly patient with advanced dementia. Her daughter often remarked that, among the team of medical professionals caring for her, I was the only doctor she liked and cooperated with. I honestly cannot say what it was I did for that to be the case. Maybe it was because she reminded me of my grandmother, and therefore I was very patient with her and connected with her as a person at each session before trying to treat her as a patient. It may have been that I visited her and examined her at her home, where she felt more comfortable. Or maybe I reminded her of her grandson. Who knows? In any case, we found a way to relate to each other and develop such a good aura and connection. That connection enabled me to deliver and her to enjoy a high level of care and satisfaction for both of us.

But it wasn't all kindness and flowery platitudes. Nelson was a seventy-six-year-old patient when I was twenty-six. He was not properly brushing or flossing his teeth. I began to lecture him about the importance of proper oral home care. Apparently, the speech went on too long. He suddenly held up his hand as a gesture for me to stop. He asked me how old I was. I said twenty-six. He said that he was seventy-six and that he still had all of his teeth, and if in fifty years when I turned seventy-six I still had as many teeth as him, I would be allowed to speak to him that way. He wasn't mean about it. He was simply giving me an understanding as to how the speech sounded from the other side of the podium. It was a great learning point. Most times, it's not what you say but rather how it is perceived.

No discussion about beloved patients is complete without the mention of Lou Sodano. Lou was one of the patients that came with the practice that I bought to start my career in 1987. He had advanced periodontal disease and several missing teeth. I restored his lower arch with a long-span multi tooth bridge. I removed several hopeless teeth, enlisted the help of an excellent periodontist, Dr. Louis Galiano, and constructed what gives me joy to say was the finest restoration of my thirty-eight-year career. It looks as good today as the day I placed it in 1988. The reason it gives me joy to say that is because Mr. Sodano has been the kindest, most soft-spoken, most appreciative patient I have ever met. No patient deserved my very best work more. There is a warmth and humble magnetism to this man that one rarely comes across. He has continually been the standard against which all patients in my practice have been measured. I have yet to meet his equal, and I am quite sure that I never will. My life has been better to have had him in it. Even when I asked him one rainy day why he was limping, he shrugged it off and asked me how I was doing. I had to find out from his son that he was wounded in World War II on D-Day, because he never uttered a complaint or any other negative word in the thirty-five years I have known him.

The Blanket

FLORENCE AND WAYNE were another older couple that also came with the practice. They were very kind, appreciative, salt-of-the-earth type of people. At one point, Florence became afflicted with cancer and was bedridden. She had lost a lot of weight, and her dentures would no longer fit. This prevented her from being able to eat and compounded the nutritional problem. Her husband came in and asked if there was anything I could do for her. They lived nearby, so I visited her at home to take a look. I tried to adjust and reline the denture, but it became evident that a new set would be better for her. Over the course of the next few weeks, I went there four or five times, taking impressions, measurements, and finally inserting the new dentures in time for Thanksgiving and Christmas dinners. Whenever I went there, she was cheerful and appreciative and usually knitting. My wife was pregnant with our first child, and Florence always asked how she was doing. My daughter was born just before Christmas, and I got caught up in my world. In mid-January, Wayne came in to tell us that Florence had passed away. He was carrying a box. As I opened the box, I found a pink-white-and-blue, hand-knitted baby blanket. Wayne explained the colors by saying that Florence didn't know whether we were having a boy or a girl. It was that blanket that she was knitting during all those visits.

That blanket remains by far the most cherished keepsake of my career. It taught me very early on just how much of an impact we can have in the lives of our patients. It taught me how much it means to people to be acknowledged and taken care of. And it taught me not for the last time how a minimal effort on our part often translates into a monumental appreciation on the part of some of our most deserving patients. That sort of emotional return on investment is immeasurable.

Another older woman, Connie, came to my practice needing quite a bit of work. I told her that some but not all of her remaining teeth should be removed by an oral surgeon and then I would make her a partial denture. She wanted them all out. I explained to her why keeping some of the teeth would be better, especially on the lower so that something more stable than a full denture could be made. Her husband agreed wholeheartedly, pointing out that he never wore the lower dentures his dentist had made for him. During the conversation, she explained that her father had died during dental surgery and that she was terrified that the same would happen to her. If she absolutely had to run that deadly gauntlet, she only wanted to do it once. I reassured her and eventually convinced her to follow my advice. A few days later, she had a 9:00 a.m appointment at the oral surgeon's office. As it was on my way into my office, I stopped in to say hi. She had only met me once, but when I walked in, you would have thought it was Jesus walking in. I only stayed about fifteen minutes, but she was so relieved to see a familiar face, a face that she trusted, that it nearly drove her to tears. All went well, and in the end, I probably ended up with about twenty-five new patients referred by her and her family.

While these two stories may be very dramatic examples, the fact is, when you go above and beyond, even very slightly, it really sets you apart. I've probably come into the office after hours only a few times a year if that. And it's usually just to get them out of pain or simply reassure them. Living near my office, it is rarely a big deal. Most times, I'm not doing anything very important, and if I am, they gladly wait an hour or two to be treated so specially.

The Lives We Connect With

OVER THE COURSE of a career, seeing these people year after year, they start to become part of us and we of them. I know that sounds a bit dramatic, but we do rub off on them and they on us. You start to feel like part of a family when you get to the point of treating five generations of that family. Five generations is a lot. We're talking about a range of people born in three different centuries. You know you're connected when you arrange for two previously unacquainted patients to meet and they invite you to their wedding a year later. You regret some of the personal connections when the sheriff's deputies show up in your office at the completion of his visit to seize a child from a parent who had violated their custody arrangements. You begin to feel like an inspirational part of their lives when a personal trainer patient of yours and one of her clients (both patients of yours) playfully and competitively bicker and ask you to judge whose flossing technique is better and who has the more robustly healthy gums. You feel a certain amount of inappropriate quiet pride when a patient who recently had you do a smile makeover with veneers gets arrested for assaulting and ramming the car of a co-worker for punching his mouth and jeopardizing my veneers. We go to their christenings and baby namings, their weddings, their shivas and funerals, and they celebrate and mourn with us as well.

The emotional availability, willingness, and in fact eagerness to connect with other people is something some people seem to be born with and some do not. If you are someone who easily connects with others, congratulations. That trait will serve you well in dentistry. If not, work on it. Sometimes "working on it" is work. Other times, it is easy and actually fun. When I was in dental school, I worked part time a few nights a week loading airplanes for a major delivery company. I met a man who had fought in the Korean War as a young paratrooper. Although he was tough as nails, Sam was dentally phobic as a result of battlefield injuries and dental treatment rendered in a MASH unit during the war. Consequently, he had not visited a dentist for over thirty-five years when I came to know him. I became friendly with him and told him that, when I became a dentist, I would take care of him. He just shrugged and in his Tennessee drawl said, "I don't know, Tom, I don't know." The crew at the airport would regularly stop at a local bar after the shift was over on Friday nights, from about 11:30 p.m. till about 1:00 a.m., to socialize and unwind. Once I became a dentist, I went to that bar at about 12:30 p.m. (after he had acquired bit of liquid courage), had a drink myself, and convinced him to come to my office and let me examine his teeth. No needle, no drills, not even an X-ray. The next week, no drink for me, and we took X-rays. The week after that, he got the most gentle cleaning possible. At that point, with trust established and phobia greatly diminished, we were able to switch to daytime appointments. Little by little, I was able to fully restore his dentition. After he retired, he moved back to Tennessee but continued to travel to New Jersey and remained a patient in my practice. I consider patient management and personal interaction to be my greatest skills as a dentist and that case to be the proudest example of that in my career.

Despite the accumulation of these anecdotes and events, we still sometimes underestimate the effect we have on these people's lives. Every once in a while, we get a reminder that hits home a little more poignantly than others.

I once had a woman in her mid-forties come in as a new patient. She actually came in because her ex-husband had been a patient and I had done a few minor things for him. Having heard only bad things about her from the ex, her reputation preceded her. At her first visit, when she did not smile or laugh at my charm or my jokes, I felt that her ex was right in his characterization of her. She certainly appeared miserable and nasty. Then she opened her mouth, and I immediately understood why she never smiled. Her teeth were discolored, chipped, and crooked. After a certain amount of cosmetic dental improvements, her teeth looked significantly better. Her confidence soared, her smile returned, and she truly seemed to be a happier person. She began to date, got a promotion at work, and referred several patients to my office.

One of the people she recommended was her sister. Also in her mid-forties but never married, she suffered from low self-esteem. She coped by being shy and sweet and never smiling. Her dental problem was mostly one of very unaesthetic malocclusion. A course of Invisalign treatment with limited but achievable realistic goals made quite a difference. She came into the office one Monday morning to tell me that she almost called my home number at midnight on Saturday. I asked, "Why; was something wrong?" She replied that she was at a wedding and a man asked her to dance and told her she had a beautiful smile. She began to cry because no one had ever told her that in her entire life.

Jimmy was a retired navy vet, fireman, and carpenter. Quiet, scruffy, and hardworking, he was liked and respected by all. He never asked anyone for anything and had a heart of gold and was always ready to help anyone else. He was tough as nails and somewhat oblivious to pain, for the most part. He only sought medical attention for wounds that duct tape wouldn't close up. But for some reason, he did keep pretty regular cleaning appointments. It may have been because, as a sailor and fireman, he understood the importance of maintenance. It may also have been due to the fact I earned his respect about ten years earlier when I spotted what turned out to be a blockage in his carotid artery that showed up on a panoramic radiograph. I referred him to a cardiologist, and he had it treated. From that point on, he told everyone that I had "saved his carotid" and prevented a stroke.

Jimmy came in about five years ago for a cleaning. He was a little overdue because he had been taking care of his elderly wife in her final days in their rural home. We asked him how he felt, and he said fine. When he opened his mouth, we could see that he was lying. As usual, he was too tough and too proud to admit pain. What I saw was the worst oral cancer I had ever seen in person or in a book. An entire section of his maxilla had been eaten away, and three or four teeth were hanging by threads. I sent digital pictures to several oral surgeons, and each said that he needed a hospital and an oncologist, not an oral surgeon. I told him to go to the hospital. He refused, saying he was fine. I insisted. He promised to go in a day or two. I made him understand how worried I was about him and pleaded that he go there on his way home as a favor to me. I called the attending oral surgeon there to be sure he would be seen. Jimmy relented, went, and they immediately admitted him. I called his son (who I had never met) and informed him of what was going on. It turned out the oral cancer was just the tip of the iceberg. His body was riddled with cancer, and the maxilla was just a distant metastasis. I visited him the next day in the hospital, and I was humbly shocked by how impressed and thankful he was with such a simple gesture as a brief visit. He was on the phone with someone when I walked in and was so proud to tell them who had come to visit him. Unfortunately, he passed away in the next week or so.

I went to the wake and was approached by a young man that I had never met face-to-face. It was the son, and he thanked me profusely for all that I had done. I said regretfully that I hadn't really been able to do anything to help his condition and wished I had seen him earlier when it might have made a difference. He shook his head and pointed out that were it not for the fact that I made Jimmy go to the hospital and moreso that I called the son, Jimmy would have gone back to his house in the woods and died alone without his son or grandchildren being able to say goodbye. Without realizing it, these are the involvements we sometimes have with people.

All You Have to Do Is Look Like You Care

THERE IS ONE thing all patients want that will set you apart from some other dentists and guarantee patient loyalty. Here it is, the golden secret. Make sure no one is reading over your shoulder, and promise not to tell anyone else! All you have to do is look like you care. That's it. And the best way to do that is to actually care. Care if you are truly helping them. Care if you are hurting them during a procedure. Care about whether they are afraid. Care about how they look and about how they feel about the way they look. Care about the quality of your work. Care about their health and well-being. Care that the treatment plan you present is right for them and is something achievable. Care about all these factors and probably a few more.

I know it seems like a lot of work and energy, but it actually comes pretty naturally after a while. The dividends it pays back both emotionally and financially are amazing. The long-term benefits of traveling on the high road like that are immeasurable. Emotional rewards are unlike financial compensation. Money paid to you is really just numbers written on small pieces of paper and deposited into bank accounts. From these bank accounts, you write numbers on other pieces of paper that you share with staff members, landlords, labs, suppliers, the IRS, and various others. In the end, you hope that there is some left over for you. But the emotional rewards are all yours and yours to keep for as long as you like. Much like the pink-and-blue baby blanket.

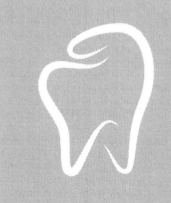

PART TWO

THE BUSINESS

The Price of Caring

THERE IS, however, a price to be paid for all this caring. To be caring or empathetic is to share the pain. If you're afraid to hurt them with the drill, you may leave decay. Fear of making them gag might lead you to not position an impression tray properly or remove it from their mouth too soon. Caring too much about their finances leads to presenting less than ideal treatment plans. Too much concern about their schedule could make you rush treatment. There certainly needs to be a limit as to how much you "care." Ultimately, your caring must center on delivering the best dental care you can with at least some awareness of those other factors.

Another negative aspect to all this caring is that you should not expect it back. It may sound whiny to point this out, but that's simply not the way it works. Some patients come to expect you to be at their beck and call. They expect discounts, extended hours, and acceptance of their tardiness and broken appointments.

This certainly does not apply to most patients. In fact, it probably seems like a bigger number than it actually is. Emotionally as well as financially, it is wise to try to build your practice around the good patients and find a way to avoid the bad ones. Forget about training the bad ones. That's one of the things that makes them bad: they can't or won't be taught.

Risk Management

AS ALLUDED to earlier, the best way to deal with trouble in life is to recognize it early and take steps to avoid it. Unfortunately, trouble comes in many shapes and sizes. Experience teaches us what to avoid, like a hot stove or a pile of excrement on the sidewalk. But troubles are like viruses. There always seem to be new ones out there. You get exposed to so many of them over the course of a career; fortunately, you seem to build a broader resistance. Your vision for spotting trouble becomes much better after having seen it before. That's about the closest you can come to immunity, but as I said, there's always new variants popping up, and some are bound to sneak past your defenses.

Sometimes it's not enough to be able to gauge whether the patient is a lunatic. Sometimes the patient is reasonably normal, but the spouse or parent is the problem. In these cases, the patient is thrilled with the care and the work that was done, and they walk out happy. An hour or a day later, the phone call comes. "My wife says they're too big" or "they're too small" or "they're not white enough."

In retrospect, this pattern is not very difficult to predict if you have met both of them, especially if you've seen them interact. If you've met the spouse and found him or her to be very critical as well as domineering, you can almost be certain that you'll get that phone call or complaint at the next visit. Sometimes, you'll even hear the troublesome spouse harping in the background. The classic example of this that I experienced was a couple that had both come in for treatment. She had porcelain veneers done at another office, which were nicely done. Yet she was extremely dissatisfied. Her complaints were irrational, and her attitude toward the previous dentist could not have been more unfounded or negative. Her toxicity was obvious and impossible to miss. I wanted no part of her and explained that they were beautifully done and that mine would be no different. The only difference is that they would be spending a great deal of money for nothing different. When the husband simply asked how much, she glared at him and angrily told him to be quiet. I noticed the daggers and managed to avoid treating her but foolishly thought he would be easier to deal with, so I agreed to treat him. Several months later, when I attempted to make him several anterior crowns, I ended up making three sets of temps before she was satisfied with the color. "Toilet bowl white" as I recall was what it took to satisfy her. He didn't return to proceed with the case for nearly five years. His white temps were now a filthy shade of brown. He was every bit as emasculated as he had been five years prior, and she remained just as unpleasant. The fact that he returned made me think that I had not done a good enough job of chasing them away. When he returned after those five years, this time I was completely unyielding in my recommendations, and I think I insulted him deeply enough to drive him away for good. There would always be problems with those two. It was the smart move to find a way to chase them out and be rid of them.

There had been several instances where this happened before I finally wised up and improved my communication of the finality of their acceptance. If they felt the spouse was going to veto it, they should bring the malcontent spouse into the office. This can certainly be phrased in nonadversarial terms, but the message needs to be conveyed. Otherwise, you will become a slave to the unreasonable demands of an unseen third party. Once the treatment goals have been established, it is always advisable to make good temporaries and get all the discrepancies ironed out as early as possible, leaving fewer chances for surprises, disappointments, and disagreements in the final product from the lab.

Parents can be just as bad. You work on a kid and do a nice job. The kid is happy and leaves. Then you get the call from Mom saying how unhappy the kid is. You feel like a terrible person for hurting a kid's self-esteem, so you get the kid back in to restore his or her confidence and make him or her happy. Usually, the kid was happy with what was done and mad at his overbearing mom for making him come back.

They teach you in dental school to instruct the parents to wait in the waiting room. In this day and age of helicopter moms and overly sensitive dads, it's a little tougher to sell that idea. But it was some of the best advice given to me, and I wish I had heeded it more consistently. First and foremost, when Mom and Dad are not around, kids are much more resilient and cooperative than we as parents give them credit for. They have been taught to follow instructions and cooperate in school already. But whenever they've come across anything they would prefer to avoid, if Mommy and/or Daddy are there to make it go away, the kid will always play that card. Oftentimes, Mommy and Daddy protect them against "threats" that they haven't even considered. Between the parents own fears and the coddling of their children's fears, it's a miracle we can ever work on a child. I always want to strangle a parent when they utter the phrase "The NEEDLE won't HURT." Another great one is "See? I told you not to eat that candy. Now you're going to get your tooth drilled!" As if the kid didn't already feel like they were being dragged up the steps to the guillotine. Thanks. By the way, who was the imbecile that made the candy available to the kid or not see to it that he brushed his teeth in the first place?

The bribe scenes are equally infuriating. The kid is misbehaving until his misbehavior earns him a bribe from the parent in order to co-operate. Is it so surprising that this invariably leads to further levels of misbehavior designed to extort an even larger reward? Ice cream gets upstaged with a toy and a toy escalates to demands for a bigger, more expensive toy. Does appeasement really ever work?

Be the Second Guy

A PATIENT CALLS and says a filling fell out. He comes in with a badly broken-down tooth and requests a new filling. Seventy-five percent of the tooth is gone, and you explain that he needs a crown or onlay. He smiles, nods, listens politely, and then says, "I want a filling." You explain again that a filling will not protect the tooth nor will it even stay in place. You explain that the reason the tooth broke and the filling came out in the first place was because the previous filling was too large and the tooth was structurally compromised. He nods understandingly and asks, "How much is a crown?" You tell him. He asks, "How much is a filling?" You tell him. He says, "I want a filling." You explain yet again that it will not work, and then he asks, "Can't you just do the filling for now?" Sometimes they try to appeal to your ego, telling you how great your work is and how it is sure to work. Or they will cringe over the fee for a crown and make you feel guilty for being so greedy.

Here is where the crucial mistake happens. If you abide by their wishes to save them money and give them the filling, two things will inevitably happen. One, the filling will fall out or fail in some other fashion as predicted. Two, they will have amnesia as to how many times you told them that it would not work, citing only how much money they paid for a filling that lasted so briefly. In an effort to salvage the relationship and prove your skills, you redo the filling. For free, of course, out of a misguided sense of honor and self-respect. The apropos phrase here is "The definition of insanity is the act of doing something over and over again and expecting a different outcome."

After the second or third futile attempt at trying to get the hopeless filling to stay, they eventually grow tired of your shoddy workmanship and the wasting of their valuable time. They leave the practice and go to another dentist. He looks at the tooth and simply says, "You need a crown." They finally start to believe that they need the crown, and the second guy is certainly not stupid enough to try yet another filling. They agree to the second guy placing a crown. Moral of the story is, it's better to be the second guy.

As a way of avoiding there being a second guy, stick to your guns, and do not let this whole scenario play out. If you lose the patient to the second guy, so what? They're a noncompliant, stubborn, manipulative, miserly patient who doesn't respect your judgment. You weren't going to keep that patient anyway. You saved yourself the aggravation and chair time as well as the tarnishing of your reputation as the guy whose fillings always fell out. And in the long run, the same scenario will play out again and again for this person as more of his gigantic fillings fall out. You're better off without him. That person will never be more than a drain on your resources, both physical and emotional.

Take a Pass

THERE ARE many times when you should reconsider undertaking a procedure. Sometimes the downside is obvious. We should all know our limitations and have a clear vision of how things really are. For example, knowing which teeth are likely to fracture during extraction and how much of a problem they will present if they do. We need to be aware of just what it will entail to finish what we set out to do if Plan A falls apart. One of the most dreaded outcomes is the fracturing of a root tip during an extraction. It will inevitably happen if you do enough extractions. The knowledge that it might happen demands that you have a contingency plan in case it does. It must be part of the decision-making process as to whether to perform the procedure or refer it out. It's not as simple as "I'm 90 percent certain I can get that tooth out without breaking it" and then grabbing the forceps and going to town. What about that other 10 percent? It is imperative to plan out all the possible scenarios that might play out if it breaks. Will it simply involve a certain amount of extra time with a root tip pick, or will a flap need to be reflected and bone removed to get it out? If it is the latter, how proficient are your flap reflecting and suturing skills? How will you repair the unexpected osseous defect? Do you have bone graft material and membranes and the expertise to place them properly? Have you explained to the patient the extra time and fee that this grafting will require? What will the long-term ramifications to the reputation of your practice be if you drift outside your strong skill set and have to struggle to make things right (or at least less terrible)? How long will the other patients on the schedule have to wait while you try to climb out of the pit you've carelessly and stupidly thrown yourself into? How likely will they be to recommend your office to others? What about the poor person suffering in your chair? Will they send their friends and family to you after that? Will they even remain in your practice? What about the embarrassment of having to send that patient to a specialist to clean up your mess? Was the fee and the ego stroke really worth risking all of that? I'm not saying that no general dentist should ever do extractions; rather, simply that we should be extremely knowledgeable and truthful with ourselves as to all of the potential pitfalls and subsequent ramifications before deciding to proceed.

While it may be the most dramatic and potentially frightening procedure we do, it's not only oral surgery that calls for a level of calculated, honest introspection. Most of the other dental specialties have specialists because of the potential for problems that come with some of the more difficult cases. This is yet another example of the importance of having a strong awareness of the places that trouble is statistically likely to lurk so you can see it coming and avoid it in the first place. That cautious learned vision is what experience and extra training gives you. Early in one's career, in the absence of a complete and accurate knowledge base and vision, extra caution and discretion should be the chosen course of action. We should all know what our limitations are. In the situation described above, unless you have removed a great number of potentially breakable teeth, you don't really know how likely that next one is to break. You don't really know exactly whether you'll be able to get it out with a root tip pick or whether you'll need to reflect a flap. Nobody really knows, not even the oral surgeons and periodontists who take teeth out all the time. But they can make a more educated guess and are more likely to be successful if things take a less than ideal turn. They are probably much better at Plan B than you are. And, quite frankly, if things do go incredibly wrong, when they are asked in court what made them think they were qualified to undertake such a difficult procedure, they will have a much better answer than you or I.

This takes us to orthodontics. Taking impressions, bonding brackets, and attaching wires is one of the easiest set of tasks in dentistry. In fact, in most orthodontic offices, these tasks are routinely delegated to assistants, not doctors. The true difficulty lies in the diagnosis of the case. Knowing what is achievable and how to get there from the onset is what it's all about. At one point in my career, I was doing some Invisalign cases. The diagnostic system I followed was a simple one. I would wait until I had accumulated a few potential cases and then bring the models to my local orthodontist, Mark Caplan, a good friend whose judgment I trust implicitly. He would look them over and say, "This group of cases is easy; I would be embarrassed to know you if you couldn't do them. They will go smoothly by the numbers. This second group is achievable but cannot be done with basic Invisalign alone and requires a deeper understanding of the prognosis of certain tooth movements." He would offer to help me with these cases. "The third group is much harder that it looks." That usually means skeletal considerations. Had I been a real orthodontist, I would have taken a cephalometric film and known how to read it and seen and understood the hidden difficulty for myself. He would then explain what the subtle details were that represented the booby traps that an untrained "orthodontist" might not see and would ultimately reduce the chance of a successful outcome. I would gladly slide the latter two sets of models across the table to him and keep the easy, predictable one, happy to have avoided the unseen pitfalls. Even the cases that he said were sort of manageable if he helped me out with them were slid across the table to him. It was a symbiotic relationship. He got a lot of cases, and I didn't get in trouble. He also got my profound gratitude and the referral of all of my conventional non-Invisalign cases.

Don't Leave Home without it

IT WAS ONCE told to me by a navy dentist that there is no such thing as a dental emergency. Either it is a true medical emergency that warrants going to the emergency room or it simply isn't an emergency. He enjoyed the luxury of practicing in the navy and was therefore somewhat immune to being sued. He also enjoyed the privilege of out-ranking most of his patients in an environment of discipline and order. Out in the real world, it doesn't always work that way. Out here, some people think that the slightest chip or twinge from a tooth constitutes an emergency that demands immediate attention from their on-call dental servant. The good news is that, in the vast majority of cases, they just need to have someone answer the phone and tell them it will be ok. In the very few times that you actually need to see them after hours in the office, they are usually immensely grateful, and it proves to be an incredible relationship builder. Wearing casual clothing to those after-hours visits hammers home the fact that you've given them your personal time and gone above and beyond even more.

Conversely, the thing that alienates patients the most is if they come to feel disregarded. It's pretty much the flip side of what I've already talked about. If you seem uncaring, inconsiderate, or dismissive, it will be very difficult to create the loyal, comfortable relationships that you need for a stable, long-term practice. You want that sort of practice because it is familiar, stable, and self-sustaining through the in-house referrals that come from such positive relationships and the year-after-year income stream that results. It's not that hard to do. Patients don't like going to a strange new dentist. Just don't mistreat them, and it's easy to keep them. Calling some patients at the end of the day if you think they might be uncomfortable is a big plus. Not returning their calls when they're having a problem is a gigantic minus.

In other words, try to always be somehow available to direct their care or simply talk them off the ledge. Ninety-nine percent of problems are easily handled if you get to them early, communicate, and show legitimate concern. That's all they really want.

It's All about Communication

WITHOUT A DOUBT, the most important cornerstone of success in all that we do, in and out of dentistry, is good communication. It connects us as human beings and dictates the way we interact. It is a force multiplier when utilized properly and the root of much evil when it is not. Communication comes in so many forms and includes listening, speaking, and unspoken body language.

It all starts with listening. And you can't really listen while you're talking. So, make them show you theirs before you show them yours. You have to make a concerted effort to truly listen. You must not only hear the words but also seek to understand the motivation and overall message the person is either effectively or ineffectively transmitting with the string of words they use. Listen to all the words that come out of their mouths and sift out the unimportant in search of the vital. If you can dissect the sentences and get deep into the core of the message that the person is trying to send, it makes it so much easier to respond efficiently and satisfy their needs and concerns. It is also important to verify that you properly understand what is being said to you and that they also understand fully what is being said to them.

All branches of the US Military use some form of the term HUA. This is an acronym for Heard, Understood, Acknowledged. It is used to serve as a verification of communication in a line of work where lives depend on the quality of effective communication.

Misinterpretation of the message can render all your efforts unsuccessful. I will sometimes pause and specifically ask a patient if they fully understand what I'm saying. And I will occasionally also interrupt them while they are speaking for clarification that I properly understand what they are trying to tell me. As much as people do not like to be interrupted, their love of truly being listened to and being understood supersedes the insult of being interrupted. Very often the message can be misunderstood. So be sure to get on the same page and truly figure out what they are trying to say. It also makes it much easier to steer the conversation onto a manageable road when you know where it is they want to go. The more they speak, the more they help you help them.

When it's my turn to speak, I will watch their face for signs of confusion. If I sense that I may have lost them, I will slow down or perhaps even backtrack so as to make sure they still completely understand. As long as they seem hungry and able to grasp what I'm saying, I will proceed with the message and the explanation. If there is defiance or a shutting down, I'll let it go. I won't preach or harass. It won't make them listen, and it certainly won't endear me to them.

An ancient philosopher once said, "A wise man knows much but says little, whereas a fool knows little and says much." I have had the privilege of meeting several very accomplished and successful individuals considered "brilliant" by their peers. The one thing they all had in common was an incredible mastery of communication and a skill of steering the conversation from what they knew and had done to what I knew and could expand their knowledge about. Once they had steered the conversation to where they wanted it to be, they were able to learn, gain, and grow. They also gained popularity by making those around them feel validated as a result of being asked their opinions. They were excellent speakers, but they were better listeners, learners, and motivators.

Speaking of listening, there was once a Canadian physician who was legendary for his diagnostic abilities. When he was asked how he did it, he simply replied, "If you want to know what is wrong with your patients, just ask them. They will tell you." Now, obviously he did not mean that they knew what their ailment was. Rather, what he was saying was that, if you properly communicated with them and listened to all the things they said, you could pick out the clues and pieces of the puzzle. Consider it a sort of "diagnostic prospecting." You simply needed to know what questions to ask and how to separate the pertinent facts from the chatter.

He was certainly not the first historical figure known to be brilliant that showed his intelligence by gathering information rather than by giving it away. Sun Tzu and Machiavelli dictated world events by learning, processing, understanding, and utilizing their understanding of human interaction. If they could do that, we certainly ought to be able to convince patients to get the dentistry they need simply by more fully understanding them and their needs and wants.

The chatter does need to be controlled, though. It is very easy to get your train of thought and progression of treatment derailed. There is a tempo and a balance of conversation that needs to be controlled by you. They will talk because they are afraid and stalling. They will talk because they want to debate or negotiate treatment. They will talk because they aren't listening to answers you've already given. And sometimes they will talk just because they are chatty. I once did a case with crowns on four upper incisors on a retired physician. An intelligent, quiet, and thoughtful man, the case went perfectly smoothly. After cementing the perfect crowns at the second visit, he remarked how nicely they came out. I told him that it was all thanks to him, and when he looked at me quizzically, I asked him if he remembered what he said while I was preparing the teeth. He did not. "Not a darned thing," I told him. Communication is a wonderful thing but so is being allowed to focus and concentrate.

Here are some other potential pitfalls to misapplied communication. As mentioned, preaching is never received well. Neither is communicating in the wrong language. What I mean by that is, if a lawyer or writer asks you to explain something, abide by his request and use your words; do not draw him a picture. Different people's minds work differently. Accordingly, if a builder, architect, or engineer can't seem to picture or envision what you are describing, then shut your mouth and draw! Most of all, if a patient tells you they are squeamish, never, never, never hand them a mirror to show them the big hole you just drilled in their tooth or show them any nasty surgical pictures, no matter how cool or informative you think they are.

Another cautionary thought is that it is best to never ask a question that you might not like the answer to. When you think about it, that could cover a lot of ground. Don't ask a chronic complainer how they like the dentures you made for them. Nobody likes dentures! You're begging for a complaint and a confrontation. Tread very carefully when asking how a very elderly parent or spouse is doing. Quite often, you will unleash a very unpleasant discussion fraught with emotion. Even simply asking someone how they are doing can be risky because they just might spend the next twenty-five minutes telling you their life history and showing you their surgical scars. Even pointing out what a beautiful sunny day it is can earn you an argument from someone with melanoma or recent cataract surgery. And let's not even start about religion or politics! Quite frankly, small talk can be dangerous and should only be attempted with extreme caution and an emergency escape plan. You will need that escape to avoid being drawn off track and running behind on your schedule when the talker begins to run amok. Having a staff member pop in and tell you Dr. So-and-So is on the phone returning your call is one such "Beam me up, Scotty" tactic. Again, borderline dishonest but sometimes necessary.

Perhaps just as important as using your ears and mind to listen to what they say, it is also very important to read their body language, their demeanor, and their response to your first few verbal overtures. Once you get a read, you can either mirror their actions or respond in another complementary way. It's kind of complicated, and we all do it automatically to some extent, but there is an art to it when it's done very well. And it is extremely powerful in a primal, invisible sort of way. I say primal because even monkeys can do it. Monkey see, monkey do.

Mirroring is simply trying to do and be what the other person is to some extent. It is "speaking their language." First, get as good a read on them as you can by observing and listening to them as deeply as you can. Hear their words. Feel the tone. Observe their mannerisms. Watch their faces, and look at their eyes. Understand their expressions. If they are loud and bold, you should dial it up a few decibels and offer a firmer handshake than usual. If they are reserved and precise, speak more carefully and express yourself in a more professional tone. Speak quietly to the timid, and joke a bit with the jokers. Don't overdo it and become condescending in the process. Learn to dance around the balance point between them and some level of personal and professional identity of your own that will blend with them and make them feel comfortable. It's a little like going to another country and attempting to speak their language. Even if you do it poorly, they will usually appreciate you trying (to some extent, until you waste too much of their time or look like an idiot). I think on some level it's a sign of respect. The more of a chameleon you can become, the more they will identify with you and the more comfortable they will be. Comfort leads to trust, and trust leads to compliance.

After your observations and mirroring have been done, it comes time to speak. A favorite piece of reconnaissance that I've always employed is to ask what they do or did for a living. Once I've put that into my mental database, it very often automatically shapes how I describe some of the dental procedures that I may be recommending. For example, let's say there is a bit of decay adjacent to an old filling. If I am speaking to a builder, I will point out that there is some rot that may have gotten under the filling and needs to be replaced with something new and solid. If it is an engineer, I might talk a little about things like structural deficiency or coefficient of thermal expansion of various materials so as to explain why there is a gap there. To a cop, I might say "I see a break in the security of that tooth, and it's my responsibility to investigate it." I might tell an attorney that it would be irresponsible for me to not rectify the situation. The list goes on and on. Gimme a profession, and I'll give you a customized script. It's not that I purposefully fabricate these scripts in order to coerce people; it's just that in order to communicate as completely and deeply as possible, I automatically get into character via an unconscious mirroring process that sees the situation in their eyes and communicates it in the language they are most fluent and comfortable in.

I know I've droned on and on about communication, but I feel the value of it cannot be overstated. Listen, understand, and be understood. See it from their perspective. Visualize what the chessboard looks like from the other side. Understand everyone's motivations, and you will always find a more direct and successful path to a solution.

Know Your Patients and Their Wants

A GREAT EXAMPLE of the value of listening to patients, understanding what they want and don't want, and using communication skills to control the narrative for the good of all goes like this: a patient comes in for a cleaning and checkup, and during the exam, you notice that they need a small filling. There is a right way and a wrong way to proceed at this point. I once had a young associate dentist working for me who simply blurted out, "You need a filling" and followed up with "You need to schedule another appointment for that." Nothing more. Not the best way to handle it.

By comparison, I would gather more information before speaking. I would check the schedule and see if there was enough time to do it then and there. Remember "count before you calculate, calculate before you plan, and plan before you act." There almost always is enough time, especially if you anesthetize them immediately and do the restoration as soon as time permits. Once I've determined that it can be done, this is when the communication mastery begins.

If I know the patient to be somewhat dental phobic, I say, "Mary, I know how nervous you get about having work done. There is a small filling that I need to do for you, and I can already see you worrying needlessly for two weeks until we can get you in. Rather than letting you go home and worrying for all that time, please let me take care of you now and get it done right away before you even get a chance to think about it. Let's put it behind you, and you can sleep like a baby tonight."

If the patient has a busy job that makes it hard for them to come in, I say to them, "John, you have a filling that needs to be done, and I know how busy you are at work and what a pain in the neck it is to get here. Let's handle it right now while you're here and clear you up dentally for the next six months."

If the patient is someone who travels a long distance to come to our office, I will say, "Bob, I know how far you travel to see us. I am grateful and flattered for the effort you make. Please let me take care of a small filling that you need while you're here and save you the trouble of coming back so that I can acknowledge and repay the effort you show by coming here."

See the difference? Three very different messages with very different verbal nuances and undertones each tailored to meet the specific needs and wants of three very different people. Each one not only virtually guaranteed to be successful but also to endear you to them further. The benefits to them have already been clearly verbalized. The benefit to you is increased production for that day, decreased administrative efforts trying to get them back in the office to get it done, and, most of all, the improved relationship-building achieved by showing them consideration in the currency and terminology most valuable to each of them.

The Body Doesn't Lie

THERE ARE many great books out there on body language. They speak about the power of body language in many interpersonal interactions. Dentistry is a face-to-face environment which is chock-full of tensions, concerns, and several other unspoken undercurrents. A strong understanding of body language can significantly tip the chances of a productive interaction in your favor. Knowing how to read the physical signals that a patient is sending you (often unconsciously) is incredibly important. If you understand these signs and know how to respond to them both verbally and via your own silent yet powerful signs, your ability to overcome many of their fears and get to know what patients are thinking will dramatically increase. You will find it easier to gain their trust, make them feel more comfortable, and ultimately be able to deliver the care they need in an environment in which they feel safe and empowered. Mastering or at least understanding these physical cues and gestures has a great impact in the building and maintaining of relationships.

A lot of it starts with an awareness of space and physicality. Personal space can quickly set the tone in an interaction. Patients are usually already a bit nervous to begin with. Getting in too close too fast can make them even more uneasy. When trying to get them to relax and engage in conversation, I will often back up to a distance of three or four feet and casually lean away from them so as to coax them out of their shell.

Placing a hand gently on an arm or a shoulder is a somewhat risky gesture. On one hand, it connotates a comforting human touch and creates a gentle connection. On the other hand, it can pretty easily be viewed as an intrusion upon someone's body or personal space. Tough call. Don't do it unless you're quite sure you've been given a green light to do so. Even then, the lighter the touch and the more brief the duration, the better. Most importantly, arms and shoulders only!

There are many physical cues described in the literature. One of the most important to utilize as a dentist is to face a patient and make eye contact as a way to demonstrate sincerity and an effort to establish rapport. Eye contact when they are speaking conveys active listening. Eye contact when you are speaking imparts a sense of honesty and trustworthiness.

Another physical cue common in our world is to gesture with open arms and upward palms as a way to show caring support and a welcoming environment. It says, "Come to me; I will take care of you." By contrast, crossed arms or palms away or down suggest a closed-minded, "Stay away!" "Not my problem" attitude. So subtle yet so potent in a visceral and unconscious way.

You Never Know Who You're Talking To

IN ORDER TO find some common ground with a new patient, a lot of times we find ourselves playing the "do you know so-and-so game." It's a much riskier game than you think. The best rule is to simply never say anything negative about anyone. It diminishes you and marks you a gossip and can only come back to you negatively. Even positive gossip and name dropping isn't always guaranteed to work out well. It's impossible to know how two people you barely know feel about each other. Speaking positively about someone who the person you're talking to hates is not going to turn out well. I know; I've done it. How was I to know? Probably best to bash no one and only speak highly of someone you know quite well and know to be universally liked. Even then, you probably want to feel the person out a bit. But by that time, you should already be building your own reputation, so don't bother.

Early in my career, I had quite a few patients who were firemen and police, both in my town as well as in surrounding towns. They all know each other, and they very often have strong opinions about each other. I had a new patient one day that happened to be a fireman. He had a very unusual name. While I was working on him during his first visit, we received a phone call. My receptionist came into the room and told me that a man with the exact name was on the phone asking for pain pills. (As a side note, miraculously, I've only gotten about three of these drug request calls over thirty-five years.) Confused by the coincidence, I looked at the fireman in the chair. He simply said, "Don't do it." I pressed him for an explanation, and he told me that this other unrelated person with the same unique name lived in the same town. This other person was constantly in trouble with the police and credit agencies and had a very serious drug problem. Over the next few years, the fireman would tell me stories of the embarrassing inconveniences of the mistaken identities. He told me that the other guy's wife also had a drug addiction problem and had been arrested for prostitution. Eventually, the fireman told me that the other man succumbed to an overdose and died. He told me that, a few months later, our town's fire department had been requested to help out at a fire in an adjacent town. While there, he noticed a large, angry, burly cop staring at his nametag. Being all too familiar with this kind of mistaken identity situation, he said, "I know what you're thinking, but I'm not him." The cop said, "I know you're not, but do you know about the wife?" The fireman briefly considered a rather disrespectful quip, but something stopped him. Turns out she was the cop's little sister.

Moral of the story . . . you never know who you're talking to, so unless you feel that the person you might reference is truly an honorable person that would be liked by anyone with a sense of right and wrong, keep your mouth shut, and don't play the "do you know so-and-so" game. Put it in the same taboo box as politics and religion. It's just not worth the risk for the sake of a measly conversation point.

Blood Money

IT'S BEEN said "their money is as green as the next guy's," but in the business of dentistry, nothing could be further from the truth. "Blood money" is a more accurate description of the income generated by your most troublesome patients. An observation has been made in business that says something to the effect of 90 percent of your business and livelihood comes from your best customers (patients) and that 90 percent of your aggravation comes from your 10 percent worst customers (patients). I agree in very broad, nonspecific strokes with this concept but would probably tweak the numbers a bit for our industry. I think that the vast majority of our patients are good people that fall in the neutral category between the best and the worst and therefore represent the biggest steady source of our income. The bulk of the practice's income comes in daily from people whom you neither love nor cringe from. These patients are the bread and butter of our practices.

It certainly seems very debatable as to what percentage of our financial rewards come from what percentage of our best patients. I do think that the emotional aspect of the equation might actually be a little easier to quantify and believe in. You could probably look at several days on the schedule or a month or even your entire patient list and count the patients you dread seeing and divide that by the total number of patients to define what percentage of your patient pool provides you with most of your aggravation versus joy. I am sure that most of the angst comes from a rather small percentage of your overall list of patients.

Ultimately, I do think that, in the long run, we can shape that percentage. In fact, the hope that I can further control that percentage as I continue to practice was one of the primary reasons for writing this book.

What Makes a Toxic Dental Patient?

OPINIONS AS to the relative importance of this topic will vary, but I present that there are several commonalities to be found. Basic rudeness and inconsideration certainly top the list. Their poor manners get in the way of a smooth performance of the duties of our staff and us. They can slow us down, make us resentful, and cause us to act reactively rather than proactively.

On a more philosophical level, toxic behavior is anything that directly prevents us from coming close to providing the unachievable goal of delivering perfection in our work. We were all tasked with that quest in dental school, where it was beaten into our hearts and minds that anything less than perfection represented sloppiness, failure, and in fact, a crime against humanity. Therefore, anything or anyone that stands in the way or hinders us in this mission is the enemy, a dental evil agent if you will. The resentment we harbor for that kind of patient as well as for lab technicians and dental assistants that chronically disappoint us weighs heavily on our psyche.

A patient that refuses or simply does not follow our treatment recommendations prevents us from providing what we honestly think is best for them. It is frustrating and to some extent condemns us to some level of failure or compromise before we even start. It also carries the insult of our opinion being diminished or disrespected. The breakdown of the trust and confidence starts there. That is the soil in which resentment, alienation, and apathy germinate and grow. But there may be many reasons why they don't proceed. These might include dental anxiety, scheduling conflicts, and, of course, money, but a slight chipping away at the enthusiasm of the relationship from our point of view certainly can result. We need to consider those other possibilities and not always take it as a personal affront. Hard as it may be to imagine, it's not always about us.

Patients that don't show up for their appointments can be very upsetting to us. We very quickly recoil against it because of the obvious financial impact and loss of revenue to our practices. I would contend that the hidden deeper emotional injury to us comes from the double whammy of business interruption and insult that this blowoff represents. Some people advocate charging for missed appointments, but the fact is that you cannot get away with charging the amount they would have paid had the appointed procedure been performed. And the money doesn't wash away the insult and the resentment.

A good friend once told me about a patient that failed to show up for a full morning appointment involving the placement of multiple implants. She called back and was given another long appointment. Again, she blew it off. He told the staff not to give her another appointment. She was furious. She wanted another appointment and said she would pay a broken-appointment fee. He said, "Fine, $12,000 is the penalty." She agreed until she found out that the 12k was a penalty and not a prepayment for the implants to be placed at another appointment. She obviously refused and went elsewhere. My friend was happy with the outcome. He chose that amount because that's what it had cost him in lost revenue due to her irresponsibility and inconsideration. She would undoubtedly continue to cost him money in future incidents. It is ridiculous to charge some measly, petty, punitive amount that doesn't come close to what their actions cost you. And it only alienates the patient and makes them feel as though they have paid for the right to disrespect you and your office. In my humble opinion, he was right to be glad to be rid of her.

Aside from the occasional large restorative cases we sometimes perform, I suppose that our financial security and prosperity and success comes from the much broader, consistent, year-after-year performance of us, our staff, and patients in general. Large restorative cases can make a profound impact on the production numbers of the month in which they are charged out. But the extra effort, time, expense, and stress that often go along with them can sometimes partially tarnish the financial glamour of them. I personally feel that there is actually more profitability and satisfaction in flawlessly, smoothly, and quickly going through small-scale focused care on a day-after-day, year-after-year basis. Doing so, we enhance and maintain the health of our patients as well as that of our practices. Our reputations, practice stability, and referral patterns certainly benefit from that.

Furthermore, I think some of these large cases are sometimes pursued for the wrong reasons. Our egos, the allure of the large fees, and more nobly, a desire to do something magnificent for a patient are all potential driving forces. But in doing so, we sometimes disregard or overlook some of the warning signs that we should all consider regarding these large cases. Things like the true cost and time required to complete them and the effect that may have on the rest of our practice all must be taken into consideration. I am in no way advocating against comprehensive dentistry. I am simply saying that it should be done for the right reasons and viewed as the serious entity that it is with a thorough understanding of all its ramifications. I am also not saying that we as GPs cannot or should not do very large cases. I would simply state that there is a time and place for a referral to a prosthodontist, and we should all know when and where that time and place is.

Pick Your Winners

EVEN THE SORT of patients that seek our care is to some extent controllable by us. Many years ago, I read an article that talked about shaping your practice to better suit your preferences. It doesn't always seem like it, but in the big picture, over time, we actually do have more control over who we treat than we think. The author of this article suggested taking a look at a list of all your patients and identifying the 5 or 10 percent of people on your list that you truly enjoy working on and how well you seem to relate to them. These preferences and criteria will likely focus on personality and character. You should also take the sort of dental procedures that these patients generally request and the value and business profitability of those procedures into account. Maybe you like to do a lot of fillings rather than large crown and bridge restorations. Or maybe you take pride in the completion of these large complex cases when planned and executed properly. Or maybe your practice is based on a large number of people coming in for regular cleanings to maintain their periodontal health year after year. Whatever it is, there are certain aspects that will make you smile and others that will make you cringe.

A pattern will become evident among these favorite patients. There will be similarities within the list. Maybe the patients in your favorite group are young, maybe they're old. Maybe there are more males versus females, fun versus serious, professionals versus blue-collar. Or vice versa on any of those choices, as well as several other variables. There will be commonalties within the group. You will have identified your ideal prototypical patient. Then do the same with 10 percent of the worst. You have now identified your prototypical antagonist patient. You can then tailor your practice around the prototypical patient you want and away from the antagonists who you do not enjoy. This will enable you to steer your practice and your life into a more controlled environment that you enjoy rather than endure. Tailoring could mean anything and everything: from the hours your practice is open, kid friendliness for moms, dads, and families versus a quieter more sophisticated environment; the way you contact your patients; the style and message of your marketing; the décor and dress code of your office; right down to your speech patterns and to some extent that of your staff as well. Cater to the needs and preferences of the type of people you want. Conversely, while I might not instigate or intentionally alienate the people from the negative groups, I certainly would not institute measures that they as a group uniquely prefer. You can't be everything to everyone, so you might as well be the best you can be to those you want to be around.

Remember, birds of a feather flock together. Once you start accumulating preferred patients, they will send likeminded people. Over the course of several years, this will lead to the development of a practice you enjoy living in rather than a prison you feel tortured within. Ultimately, you and your staff will thrive in a more productive and profitable, comfortable and inspiring environment.

Suicide Mission

SOMETIMES, a patient walks in, and you do your records-gathering and data collection. You listen to what the patient wants and try to picture the feasibility of achieving those goals. If you have done this a few times, you can envision multiple pathways and outcomes. This is especially true on the more complex cases. The prognosis of these potential results depends on many things: patient cooperation in terms of availability for the required number of visits, patient's compliance in specialist's offices, operator skill set, as well as that of the specialists and dedication of all involved come into play.

Finances are very often a limiting factor. This one comes in a variety of forms. Sometimes it's as simple as what the person can afford. Dentistry can be very expensive, and not everyone has enough money. More often, it boils down to what they can justify. That is a reflection of the value that they place on their dental health and the things we do for them. That can be shaped by how they were raised, how thrifty they are, and how much they connect their dental health to their overall health. Psychological issues like fear of losing their teeth and how that is connected to aging can affect the value placement and decision-making. With regard to the aesthetic ramifications, people will always pay more for what they want than for what they need. A great example is how quickly patients will pay $500 for whitening but balk at $100 for diagnostic X-rays. Different people have different motivators. I am not advocating the identification of these motivators as a means to "sell" them dentistry; rather, it's a means to try to understand their wishes and do the best you can to help them achieve their individual goals while, hopefully, simultaneously doing what you consider best for their dental and overall health. Their reason and your reason do not have to be the same as long as the final result achieves both criteria.

A perfect example of this is adult orthodontics. I look at an adult with crooked teeth, and I worry about the lack of cleansability and subsequent periodontal disease. I also worry about the long-term ramifications of wear and tear on the teeth, bone, and periodontium as a result of the malocclusion. So, I recommend orthodontics. They agree to proceed with it. Not because of the perio or the occlusion. They agree because of the aesthetics. I don't care why they agree, as long as they agree.

Sometimes, in the diagnosis and treatment planning of a complex case to help a patient, you may miss or not properly factor in some of the warning signs that can signal the potential for difficulties en route to the result that you and/or your patient would like to envision. Some of these complications might include less-than-optimum periodontal health and home care. Sub-optimum bone quality and/or quantity could be an issue. Improper tooth positions or angulations can bring more trouble than you might think. Badly placed implants can often greatly diminish the possibility of a good outcome. For reasons of philanthropy, ego, or simple ignorance, you may find yourself deaf to the voices of reason coming from specialists or your own knowledge base. You disregard these warning signs, and you forge on forward, against sound advice, convinced that, if you simply give it your best, maybe you can make it work. Sometimes you can. Perhaps it just takes a little more chair time. Maybe it just costs a few more dollars in lab and supply costs than usual. Even these two less-than-catastrophic scenarios can erase profitability in amazingly short order, and you can only afford to indulge yourself in these expeditions occasionally. Sometimes, it's worse. It takes more time. Much more time. And costs more. Significantly more. But the worst part of it is that, deep down, you come to realize that you are in a no-win situation. A failure that you should have seen coming but chose to ignore the potential pitfalls of. This case has no chance of ending up the way you wanted (and promised) it to. You're on a road that you know ends in disappointment. A costly road with no exit, that you wish you never took, that ends in frustration, anger, embarrassment, and regret. You hate yourself for ignoring the warning signs and vow that you will never go down a road like this again. But as the old saying goes, "The road to hell is paved with good intentions," and it is likely that you haven't taken your last walk down that road.

The only avoidance I can see to traveling on this road is to get better at remembering how these things usually play out and not kid yourself into thinking that it might be different this time. You need to become an expert in reading not only the dental components of it but also all the interpersonal ramifications mentioned above. And if you must embark upon that road, proper communication of the difference between the realistic outcomes versus their imagined outcomes must be clearly expressed and documented at the very onset of this risky endeavor. Remember, it's an explanation before, and an excuse after the fact. It still won't be fun, but at least you might be able to mitigate some of the costs and hardships. Or at least not look and feel like so much of a failure.

The Price of Beauty

THE PREVIOUS chapter opens up the discussion of cosmetic dentistry and some of its ups and downs. Giving it its own name and implying that it is a specialty is a bit misleading. Everything we do has a certain amount of aesthetic dentistry involved. Even a silver filling on the farthest tooth back in the mouth is sculpted to try to make it look nice. A partial denture with metal clasps on it should still have aesthetically pleasing denture teeth and pink acrylic made to look as natural as possible. A simple prophylaxis that includes the polishing away of unsightly stains from the teeth and makes the gums more beautifully healthy increases the aesthetic value of a smile and could be called cosmetic dentistry.

When people use the phrase "cosmetic dentistry," I suppose they are talking about procedures done solely for aesthetic purposes rather than tooth repair or replacement. These cases can be incredibly rewarding in terms of the increased self-esteem and confidence we can give to people. It can be exhilarating to create beauty where it was previously missing. These cases can be financially profitable because, as mentioned, people will pay for what they want more readily than for what they need.

However, these cases can be tricky business for several reasons. First off, one must get used to the idea of sometimes destroying healthy tooth structure. It always feels a little wrong and treads very close to running afoul of our oath of "Do no harm." But we justify it as a necessary evil in the pursuit of the greater good in the satisfying of the patient's wishes and self-esteem. However, patients' wishes in this arena can be very emotional and sometimes irrational. Things like body dysmorphia disorders will guarantee that whatever you provide will not bring them happiness. A thorough, frank, and honest discussion with the patient regarding exactly what it is that they are looking for and exactly what it is that you will be able to provide is essential. You must be absolutely sure that both parties are reading from the same page before you touch that very first tooth. I once had a patient bring in a fashion magazine and show me a picture of an absolutely perfect smile on a model's absolutely perfect face and asked me for a guarantee. I told her the only guarantee I could safely give was that her smile would not be as perfect as the one in the magazine. It is always best to under-promise and overdeliver.

A crucial component of almost all cases is to recognize the potential challenges and subsequent limitations. Every case has them. Maybe it's the skeletal relation of the jaws. Or maybe the patient may have a significantly uneven occlusal or incisal plane. Gingival margin discrepancies and a high lip line can also cause your beautiful laminates to fail to electrify a smile as much as they would against a more ideal backdrop. Facial asymmetry will be very difficult to overcome, and may or may not be something that prettier teeth can help with. It's important to recognize these challenges and either have a good plan as to how to deal with them or be ready to settle for a limited, maybe even compromised result. These limitations, extra orthodontic and/or surgical procedures, and potential compromised outcomes need to be clearly and thoroughly explained to the patient before you begin. You must be sure that they completely understand and agree to the lack of a "guaranteed" delivery of what their personal imagination envisions to be a perfect smile. A deep understanding of the concept of "realistic treatment goals" is essential for all involved parties.

Even with the precautions in place, be ready to redo some of these. If not for the satisfaction of your patient, then for your own. They can become a challenge, a torment, and a labor of love as you chase an aesthetic ideal.

Many years ago, I had the pleasure to hear Dr. Gerard Chiche speak. He told us about a very demanding patient who had a smile makeover done in Texas with some very specific requests regarding tooth color and position as well as the aesthetic appearance of her gums. She wanted them straight, white, and beautiful. She was very disappointed with the results. So she flew to New Orleans to have Dr. Chiche redo the case. He showed us the Texas results, and, quite frankly, it wasn't that bad. Dr. Chiche listened to her complaints and took an approach more along her stated preferences. He then showed us his results. It was very impressive, significantly more beautiful than the previous dentist had achieved. In the opinion of every dentist in the audience, it appeared well worth the effort she put in to get it. He told us how he puffed out his chest and braced for the applause as he handed her a mirror. She looked at the beautiful natural esthetics crafted by an artistic ceramist and said "This is not what I wanted. I want my teeth to be perfect!" Most of us in the audience cringed and were horrified and glad that patient hadn't come to us.

To satisfy this demanding patient, he redid the case, and despite the mutual frustration of course, he sensed that she was not irrational and sincerely trusted him. With a great speaker's flair and a charming French accent, he explained to us that he had to satisfy her even though he was so puzzled that the patient did not appreciate the tremendous improvement over her initial situation and was not exactly sure how to plan the new design. He told us that he chose an extremely white shade contrary to his own taste and utilized the shape of the crowns to align the teeth perfectly without any irregularity whatsoever.

Then he showed us his final result. It was magnificent! In comparison, it made his first case look not so dissimilar to the Texas result. She had been right.

There are several lessons to be learned here. First, even the very best clinicians do not always achieve perfection on the first attempt at a case. Second, we sometimes do our most impressive work when pushed by our most demanding patients. But the third and most important lesson here is to recognize that, as good as something is, it can always be made better. Maybe that was the attitude those sadistic dental school instructors were trying to beat into us when they told us nothing was good enough. The point of the pencil can always get a little sharper. It may be that achieving that next level is too costly or difficult for our patients and not even something they can appreciate or care about, but we need to be aware of what can be done. We need to aspire for and be able to deliver that next level whenever the situation calls for it.

No One Wants Brown Teeth

ONE OF THE most challenging things we do is choosing a shade of porcelain for crowns to be made at the lab. Color perception is subjective to some degree. Lighting is inherently and exasperatingly inconsistent. The coloring of a tooth could not be further from monochromatic. There is always some level of a color gradient from the gum line to the incisal edge. That gradient is nonlinear and irregular. It is also inherently 3D, with the color being developed from within, at multiple depths, from multiple sources and for multiple reasons. Pulpal status often plays a part. Variations in intrinsic dentin and enamel color can produce a myriad of perceived color. Internal stains from previous restorations and/or developmental anomalies frequently leave their mark. External staining and various degrees of enamel translucency versus opacity all contribute to variations in the perceived color of teeth. The position and angulation within the mouth that the tooth sits in and how illuminated it gets affect how the tooth appears to the eye relative to its neighbors. Thus, it is impossible to truly achieve a perfect match. It simply boils down to how close you can get and how much of a compromise you and your patient can live with. That will vary from patient to patient and tooth to tooth.

As a result of these complexities, the hardest task in dentistry is to treat one of the maxillary central incisors and not the other and try to get them to match. It puts you between a rock and a hard place. It forces you to decide which rule you have to break. The rule is that the two upper central incisors must match each other. Often, this leads to treating both centrals together. Hopefully, that doesn't lead to breaking the other rule of doing no harm. It's a lot easier to justify if the innocent other central already has a crown or large fillings. If you have a high-quality lab nearby that offers shade matching if your patient goes there, I would highly recommend it for some of these situations in order to boost your odds a bit without having to sacrifice the innocent other central.

Either way, the centrals must match. They are right out there, for all the world to see. The stars of the show we call a smile. They must be identical! In study after study, the thing that is most associated with attractiveness is facial symmetry. It is biologically hardwired into us. It has been postulated that this is because asymmetry is sometimes a result of illness or genetic defect. And from an evolutionary standpoint, defects are to be avoided. We as dentists can't overhaul a person's entire attractiveness or dictate their evolutionary success, but the least we can do for them is to literally start at the middle and try to make those two teeth match.

The further back in the mouth, the less crucial it becomes. With the posterior teeth, it's usually best to err on the lighter side. They are usually less illuminated in function and may appear darker. You can always send it back to the lab to tint it a bit darker, or you can simply give the patient a whitening kit to lighten the other teeth. They'll love you for it, and their perception will accommodate. Besides, no one likes to be told that their teeth are brown.

If You Don't Know Where You're Going, Any Road Will Take You

THERE ARE several age-old sayings in business and in life. Two that seem to really pertain to dentistry are "If you don't know where you're going, any road will take you," and "Those that fail to plan, plan to fail." Both apply to the planning and running of a successful dental practice and career. It is never too early to start to visualize your goals and start to take the steps necessary to achieve them. Some of the plans you will need to start formulating will involve deciding on the size and type of practice that suits you and deciding what sort of dentistry you want to do.

When it comes to choosing the type of practice, it turns out that there are many different types of practices within the broad scope of general dentistry. There are numerous choices that we must make. Some of these choices should be made at the onset of our careers. Unfortunately, most of us are taught virtually nothing about this while in dental school. You may not need to firmly decide on these issues while you're simply trying to meet your requirements, pass your boards, and somehow escape from the hell they call dental school, but you probably should start to envision the sort of professional life ahead of you that you would like so that you will be a little more prepared to decide once the time comes. Since many recent grads start out as associates in established practices that they sometimes become entrenched in, it's important to be very honest with yourself about whether you want that to be where you end up. Financial constraints and a desire to get into the game and prove themselves often cause young dentists to grab the first job available to them. It is essential that they do not let their first several years fly by without firm commitments and plans. If you have developed an idea of what you would like your life as a dentist to be and the first place you get a job doesn't quite fit the bill, don't waste too much of your career on a path that ultimately drags you away from the direction you would like to take. Find a position in a practice whose philosophies are more compatible with yours, and start building your future earlier.

There are many choices and variables when it comes to different styles and types of practices. These choices include but are certainly not limited to:

Geographically speaking, where would you like to live? City or country, near where you grew up or far away? Once you have invested time and effort putting down roots, dentistry is not a career that generally travels well. This is because much of your value as a dentist rides on the quality of the relationships you have developed over the years with your patients. To up and leave and start all over elsewhere is to erase some of that value.

Will you work alone, or will you have a partner and/or an associate? Volumes could be written on this topic alone. Concepts like individuality versus comradery lie at the core of this decision. Having dual coverage for the practice and less financial outlay are very nice. Having zones of disparity and disagreement develop over time are not. Is it "safety in numbers" or "does not play well with others"? It really depends on two perfect partners finding each other.

Will it be a large practice with many operatories or a smaller, more intimate, traditional setup?

How insurance dependent will you be?

How many employees will you have, and how well will they be compensated relative to others in the industry?

Will you focus on new patient acquisition via marketing? Or will you participate with a broad range of insurance plans so as to fill the office? How heavily will you rely on patient retention via loyalty driven methods and systems, like internal marketing? Will you strive to encourage patient referrals and develop an active recall protocol designed to keep many of your existing patients in the fold and excited to be part of your practice?

Will your focus be heavily on restorative dentistry and refer most of the other things out to specialists, or do you intend to delve a bit deeper into endodontic, orthodontic, surgical, pediatric, and periodontal cases you feel comfortable, capable, and enthusiastic about doing?

How many hours would you like to work to achieve the balance in your life you would prefer?

How many hours do you need to work to pay for the life you would prefer?

How many patients would it take to help you achieve your financial goals? How many would it take to achieve the goals if you add an associate or share with a partner?

What type of patients would you like to treat? Blue-collar, down-to-earth people that call you doctor and place you on a pedestal but sometimes cannot afford premium dentistry, or a wealthier, more critical clientele that calls you by your first name and likes to debate the specifics of your recommendations and sometimes feel a bit more entitled in many aspects of their relationship with you?

Will you pursue and cater to young energetic patients with busy lives and priorities that sometimes come before obligations to you and the treatment you are trying to provide or older patients with a bit more time on their hands and more need for your services?

These are only a few of the options a practice owner must decide between. In fact, these previous two pages ask far more questions than they answer. But they are all important variables to be considered as you plan your career and life. Each one of these topics has several subtopics attached to them that all beg lengthy discussion.

None of them are right, and none of them are wrong. But you have to develop a philosophy and stick to it. And you have to fully understand the ramifications of each of these choices. You must put aside all your ego, preconceptions, prejudices, unfounded assumptions, and secondary motivations when you ask yourself those questions. Ultimately, the answers to these questions are opinions, and they will vary from person to person. That's the beauty of it.

You must also understand that some of the choices from some of the categories don't necessarily blend well with some of the choices you make in other categories. Another problem is when a choice is chosen but not committed to. One such contradiction would be to choose a large facility designed to handle and treat far more patients than you currently have and then not commit fully to the marketing that it will take to fill all of those chairs. Small, personal boutique practices without huge marketing budgets go better with smaller, less heavily staffed practices. The point is the combination of the choices must all work together like a proper ensemble with all the proper accessories.

Cowboy boots, jeans, a rugged shirt, a cowboy hat, and a very firm handshake is a great combination. So is a tuxedo, shiny shoes, a custom-tailored shirt with cufflinks, a manicure, and a Rolex. But the parts are not interchangeable. Pick one set, it'll work. Don't drive a muddy pickup truck to your job as the maître d' at the finest restaurant in the city or a Mercedes coupe to the feed lot to pick up tools for the care of the livestock on your large ranch. And don't ever make the assumption that the guy in the tuxedo automatically is wealthier than the guy in the jeans.

Navigating your way through all these choices is not an easy thing. It is complicated, and we haven't even started talking about what sort of services you will provide. Surgery seems exciting and rewarding until you get in over your head and find yourself in a very stressful and perhaps litigious situation. Endo seems like easy money until you factor in the need for 100 percent anesthesia, the potential for post-operative discomfort and complaints, and the bi-annual disappointment of having to look at an endodontic fill that may be a millimeter or so short for the rest of your years with that patient. Pediatric dentistry can be fun. Right up until it isn't. A little perio perhaps? Not much fun when the patient does not follow-up with the recommended home care and office maintenance and declares your therapy a failure after five floss-less years of personal neglect. How about ortho? How about they never wear their retainers and everything relapses. Again, your fault.

The point of this diatribe is not to complain about patients or the work we do. I am immensely grateful to do what I do for a living for the people in my practice. Rather, it is to urge you to fully understand all that comes with the choices we make as to what to do and what to refer out. Become very knowledgeable as to what makes one extraction, root canal therapy, pediatric dental patient, orthodontic, or periodontal case easy, manageable, and predictable compared to those that are more likely going to bring the potential for problems. Learn to pick your battles. Become a lover of the low-hanging fruit or at least the fruit that you are truly qualified to reach. Life is a constant balance of calculating risk versus reward, and dentistry has more than its fair share of those assessments. The examples are endless. Even some of the decisions as to how to proceed with some of the procedures that we are eminently qualified to do beg some consideration. Choosing to start an elective crown and bridge restoration on a patient who is going away on a trip for a while, where you will not be able to properly support him should any complication arise like sensitivity, a loose temp, or a bite adjustment, is a decision I personally would question. I still chuckle about the millisecond it took me to refuse the desperate request by a very high-maintenance patient for me to start a large porcelain veneer case ten days before her daughter's wedding. Always think about the big picture.

When in Doubt, Send It Out

NEVER LET greed or ego cloud your judgment. Don't focus on the instant fees that can be generated by doing some of the higher-risk treatments instead of referring to a qualified specialist. If you choose to take on a case that may be just outside the realm of where you excel and the patient leaves the practice because of an unfavorable outcome, you'll have to factor in the cost of losing the thousands of dollars associated with all of the future restorative and preventative treatment for a patient and their family and all future referrals because things didn't go as they would have in a qualified specialist's office. Even if the same problems happen in the specialist's office, it is perceived that it was either a very difficult case or the specialist was at fault. Either way, it's not your fault. (Except if you were the one that recommended that specialist; we'll talk about that in a bit.) You should also factor the stress and anxiety that comes in when things are not proceeding ideally. All that loss for something you should have recognized as a questionable situation from the start doesn't seem smart to me.

The last and certainly not least important reason for referring cases to a specialist is one of professional liability. While the meaning of the term "standard of care" is often vague and argued (usually by attorneys in a malpractice case), the truth is that a large percentage of dental malpractice cases are centered on a general dentist's failure to recognize difficulty and refer to a specialist when indicated. Consider the potential financial ramifications of a lawsuit if you drift outside of your lane and make a mistake. Even with malpractice insurance, the loss of time and the impact on your psyche can be enormous.

Now that I have made a strong case for referring to specialists, it is also critical that you refer to the correct specialist. The whole idea of referring someone to a specialist is that you want the patient to receive better or more predictable care than you feel you could consistently provide. You want them to have the best care possible, don't you? Therefore, once you have decided to send them to a specialist, you should make sure you recommend them to the best person possible within that specialty. That person should be skilled, compassionate, honorable, and have your patient's best interests at heart. If they do not, as the person who made the recommendation, you will find yourself sharing some of the blame for the transgressions of these sub-optimal specialists. The only thing worse than having to apologize for what you do is to have to apologize for what others do.

Early in my career, I sent several patients to an established orthodontist in a nearby town. Liked and respected in the local dental society, he was somewhat of an elder statesman. It seemed safe sending my patients to him. The problem was that, as it turned out, most of his career was spent in the sixties and seventies before implants became available. The concept of the creation of adequate space between the roots of teeth for the planned implants as well as the necessary bone around them seemed foreign to him. In his mind, as long as the stone models looked pretty, the case was a success. On two cases, the braces were taken off without my consent, with four millimeters of bone between the central incisor and canine roots even after I told him that my periodontist needed seven millimeters to have enough room to safely place an implant. His answer was that there was seven millimeters between the crowns of those teeth. He was oblivious to the fact that without enough space *between the roots*, implants could not be safely placed. Thirty years later, those two now not-so-young men are still regular patients. One has a Maryland bridge, and the other wears a partial. I know I should get past it, but my regret resurfaces every time I see them. As the next year or two went on, I came to realize that this orthodontist was past his prime. His cases were subpar. There was nothing I could do other than find someone else to refer future patients to, but I was unable to redirect the patients that were already in the course of treatment with him. I had to just watch it unfold and hope that some of my future requests would be heeded.

As my career progressed, I became a bit more discerning as to who I entrusted the care of my patients to. Good communication and perceived like-mindedness usually helped to put me into habitual working relationships with practitioners that I was able to work effectively with. My instinct usually served me well. Usually, but not always. Unlike other friendships and acquaintances where character flaws, mistakes, and digressions should be overlooked, forgiven, and the benefit of the doubt given, specialists and professional relationships should be constantly reexamined and reevaluated. Because it doesn't matter how nice the first five cases that a specialist treated seemed to be if their work or attitude toward your patients takes a turn for the worse. If you are going to continue to put your stamp of approval on someone else's efforts, you should continue to critically evaluate that person's efforts, results, motivations, and character. To ignore warning signs and continue to refer to someone whose efforts, motivations, and results start to deviate from the ideal is a very bad thing. Maybe they changed, or maybe your initial assessment of them was not critical enough and they were always subpar and you simply didn't see it. In any case, once spotted, you must react. To delay a course correction only makes matters worse. The longer it takes you to make that correction, the more the bodies will pile up. Be demanding on behalf of your patients, and be very aware of what was done versus what could have and should have been done. Patterns will emerge. A leopard's spots become easier to see once you've noticed the first few. If you notice such a change, you should be quick to make adjustments and assure proper treatment for the future patients you will refer out. Weed out specialists who do not share your level of commitment to your patients. We owe that to our patients as well as to our profession. Certain things like poor orthodontic results, unsuccessful periodontal surgeries, and carelessly placed implants are the gifts that keep on giving, compromising all restorative efforts that follow and damaging your relationship with your patients for sending them there in the first place. Being known to work closely with someone with known questionable ethics reflects poorly on you. So be sure to not only put forth your best efforts but also align yourself with others that also do so.

The choice to undertake a course of treatment or not also extends into the realm of restorative dentistry as well. Just because a patient wants a certain procedure done doesn't mean you should do it, especially if you feel that it is not in the patient's best interest or if you feel that there is not a good prognosis associated with that treatment. Poorly placed implants dropped on our restorative doorsteps seem to be an all too frequent unpleasant occurrence. It was explained to me by a prosthodontist once that, unless you're comfortable with the title of "co-defendant," do not try to place a restoration on an implant that a periodontist or oral surgeon had carelessly placed at a terrible angle in an inaccessible place with no chance of providing any usable occlusion. Unfortunately, refusal to restore something like that will always lead to an uncomfortable conversation with the patient and the specialist. But sometimes, you need to do it. All you can do is assess the prognosis of further treatment. What the patient had already spent and gone through is unfortunate, but you can do nothing about that. It is now your responsibility to not add expense, discomfort, and disappointment to the patient and implicate yourself embarking on a path with very minimal chance of a favorable outcome. As healthcare providers, it is always our first intent to help, but we need to remain aware of what will and will not work. Cases like that *will* fail through no fault of yours, yet you will share the blame and the shame in the process. Sometimes, the smart play is to take a pass.

Know Your Numbers

ASSIGNING an arbitrary number to the size of a practice you would like is meaningless without considering factors that affect the way you would like to practice and be productive and fulfilled. It is much better to give yourself a plan to follow by first establishing a practice philosophy and directional goals. Ask yourself some questions, like what level of hygiene department compliance you will devote your efforts to developing, what sort of procedures you intend (and have the opportunity) to do versus refer out, how many hours per week you would like to work, and how much delegation of duties to support staff you feel is appropriate.

It is probably wise to set those as well as a few other secondary parameters first and let the head count grow to fill it. You'll know when you've reached capacity and can adjust accordingly. This way, you can let your practice support your life and preferences rather than the other way around.

It will probably be somewhat of a sliding scale over the course of your career, with you accommodating the needs of the practice a bit more as you build it and accommodating you and your lifestyle later.

A strong sense of pragmatic business sense is essential to financially thrive in business. We are simultaneously fortunate and unfortunate to possess the ability to be highly compensated just for possessing the skills and degree obtained in dental school. What I mean by that is we can afford (to some extent) to make foolish business decisions by virtue of the fact that our income is higher than most. It seems unfortunate to have to settle for less than ideal returns on our efforts and investments. Business decisions regarding your return on investment should be determined before investing in expensive equipment, technology, or physical space. I'm certainly not advising against investing. Quite the opposite. You do need to stay current in order to inspire your patients and staff. Just beware of opinions from biased sources like salespeople with a vested interest in you buying from them. They are not bad people. It's simply their job to influence you. Many times, they believe so deeply in their product that they're being very honest in their efforts to get you to buy. Subjective variables like "wow factor" or "fun" or "personal fulfillment" shouldn't be ignored, but they should always be considered secondarily relative to sound business strategies and honest data analysis. It's always best to also seek sound financial advice from accountants and financial advisors when making these large elective purchases. They tend to be more pragmatic and are better versed in business concepts like return on investment. They rely more heavily on the numbers, and numbers don't lie.

Don't S*** Where You Eat

SPEAKING OF honesty, the phenomenon of dentists having affairs with staff that work in their offices is so common that it is almost a cliché. The combination of close quarters, wealth, the prestige of the dentist, and admiration for what is being done certainly fuels the attraction. There may even be a bit of competition on the part of some employees for the attention of the dentist, further fueling the fire.

These affairs are a terrible idea. The financial ramifications can be devastating to the practice. Sometimes the most benign of relationships or even comments or gestures in today's environment can trigger sexual harassment lawsuits. The best advice is to behave yourself and don't do or say anything you wouldn't do if your grandmother was watching.

Regarding married couples working together in dental practices, I suppose those marriages are no more or less statistically doomed nor successful than most. A positive aspect of these arrangements is that both partners share a common goal of success at the office working side by side. Additionally, the non-dentist spouse gets to see firsthand what it is that sends their spouse home drained some days. What they have going against them is the drama that often goes along when the spouse of the dentist works in the office. It often sets up a superiority/inferiority dynamic with the other staff members that is usually not good. Jealousy on the part of the spouse regarding any attention shown to staff or patients by the dentist is also often a source of marital discord, which can spill over into the practice, reducing morale and productivity. The concept of "absence makes the heart grow fonder" can also ring true compared to a couple that spends twenty-four stressful hours per day together.

As it pertains to extramarital affairs with patients, these things happen for the same reasons mentioned above and are obviously a terrible idea. It can be easy to slide into given the financial image, nurturing aspect, and most of all the fact that everyone is on their very best behavior. These affairs are not inherently built upon anything real or substantial and are poisonous to the practice. An implied sort of blackmail can corrupt the freedom of the dentist and taint the character, tone, and reputation of the practice. Again, behave!

Staff: The Best of Times, The Worst of Times

IF THERE IS anything more important to the health, strength, and success of a dental practice as the relationship between us and our patients, it is the relationships we have with the people with whom we work every day. We cannot do the things we do without an effective support staff. Keeping this staff happy is essential to staying productive. The various intertwining relationships of all those involved can be very complex and can either lead to a cohesive, cooperative, mutually supportive team or a spiteful, dysfunctional drama. At the first office I worked in, I saw a rather entitled, established, chairside assistant verbally bully a new assistant to the point that the new assistant pushed her against the wall and put a handful of sharp instruments to her throat. It certainly seems that this level of volatility should have been picked up on at the screening process of the new assistant. For that matter, the domineering attitude of the senior assistant should also have been addressed and corrected at some point in time. The owner dentist should have taken a more aware and active role in the maintenance of the interpersonal interactions between the staff members. Letting them "settle it themselves" and establish a pecking order on their own is simply not a good idea.

I bought my practice from a dentist in his seventies. The practice had not changed in many years. I kept his office manager on for the sake of continuity of the practice. She was not incredibly organized and was rather set in her ways. At one point, I hired a new assistant. She was energetic, cheerful, and full of new ideas. When I came back from lunch one day, the assistant was gone. I asked the office manager where she was, and she simply shrugged. It turns out that after I left for lunch, she screamed at the assistant who, while the office manager was away on vacation the previous week, had the audacity to reorganize the sloppy environment that had always been the norm. This infuriated the office manager. According to the new girl, I believe her exact words were "Listen, girly, I've seen silly little bitches like you come and go, so get out!" The young girl got out and never came back. Not firing the office manager was probably the first mistake of my career. But it wouldn't be the last!

Personalities sometimes collide a bit in such close confines like a dental office. It seems to be unavoidable, and it can be a shifting landscape. It is human nature, and it is unavoidable. There are certain troublesome patterns that can develop due to the structure, workflow, and compensation of a dental practice. The assistant and the doctor develop a certain bond because the doctor relies so heavily on the assistant and spends so much one-on-one time with the assistant. The doctor looks to the assistant to maintain the doctor's spirit, to help fend off negativity from the patients, and to physically assist in the delivery of care and the expression of his art. The assistant is at the point of the spear with the doctor. Ultimately, the doctor sees the assistant as a comrade in arms and seems to grant the assistant extra leeway. This can unfortunately also earn the assistant some resentment from others in the practice.

Another potential negative dynamic that can arise from the close interaction between doctor and assistant is that production can vary widely based on the mood and whims of either person. With positivity from the assistant, the doctor's production can soar. Perceived negativity from the assistant might infect the doctor, and productivity will likely suffer.

The hygienists are the talent. They are skilled, educated, and highly paid. The good ones are the co-stars of the practice and earn every penny they make by doing a difficult job over and over again with compassion, professionalism, and charm. The doctor understands this and pays them accordingly. One risk with them is that their higher level of compensation combined with occasional need for help from lower-paid auxiliaries can sometimes instigate feelings of resentment from others in the staff.

Then comes the office managers. They are the brains of the outfit. They are the ones that make the machine run and actually get everyone paid. They get the authority and the intellectual validation but can sometimes feel alienated from the clinical staff members, like military support staff members might feel when battle troops return to base after a fight.

The best you can do is to be aware of these dynamics and make an effort to minimize the more negative patterns that will inevitable arise on occasion. Not everyone has to be best friends with everyone else, but they do need to respect each other so as to form a cohesive, productive team. As the boss, it's generally best to maintain certain emotional boundaries between you and your staff. Along those same lines, employee/employer situations among friends are not usually a very good idea. In the first year or two of my career, there was an architect in a nearby office. He was in his seventies and was successful but quite cranky. He had only one employee, and they worked side by side for over twenty-five years in one large room. I once asked him what his employee's son's name was. He shrugged and said, "I dunno, Doc. Do yourself a favor and don't get too personal with your employees." Now, he may have taken that position a bit too far, but the concept is sound. You want to have pleasant interpersonal experiences with the important people around you, but at some point, familiarity breeds contempt. A balance needs to be struck because most often it is the employer who finds his hands tied with the strings of guilt and obligation once the line between friend and employee gets blurry. It is better to build a team based on professionalism, mutual respect, and goal achievement that can give everyone a sense of fulfillment and a sense of pride about the good work done for the patients in the practice.

The building and maintenance of such a team is not easy and certainly does not happen by accident. There are a multitude of human emotions and interactions that, once soured, can get in the way. Burnout and interpersonal friction can cause breakdown of the dynamics of a dental office team. A few of the things that can ensue once the organization begins to break down are as follows:

Front desk personnel can become less effective and diligent at scheduling patients and creating the opportunity for production. They are the first contact with a patient on the phone as well as the person who handles the often delicate and unenviable but essential business of collecting payment from the patients. Their face is the first face encountered when a patient enters our office and can therefore set the tone of the visit. They are the ones with their finger on the pulse of the practice. If they are not upbeat and smart, the practice will certainly not live up to its potential.

Hygienists might become less enthusiastic about motivating patients to seek and maintain the best oral health possible. Their enthusiasm is infectious to the patients and that energy level very often shapes the way people see your office and the way they feel about dentistry in general. Your hygienists spend more time with most of the patients than anyone else in the practice and have more opportunity to spread your message and set that tone. A great deal of practice loyalty is built upon the relationships forged as a result of the way the hygienists present themselves and care for the patients.

Patients can absolutely sense these elements in the atmosphere of a dental practice. Maybe it's because they spend extended periods of time with us when they cannot speak and can only observe. Or maybe their fight-or-flight antennae are up and they are therefore more cognizant and analytical of what's going on around them. It's not like a convenience store that they are only in for a minute or two and generally do not have many interpersonal relationships to observe, analyze, or care about. Needless to say, patients are usually nervous enough going to the dentist. They want to be in a happy place where everything is positive and nonthreatening. Who doesn't? Especially in a place where the potential to feel uncomfortable seems omnipresent. The last thing they want is an angry dental professional working on them. They can and will be either elevated by a positive aura or driven down by negativity. They will not be inclined to stay in a practice filled with a high tension level that makes them uncomfortable, and they certainly will not refer friends and family to a place like that.

When the interpersonal connections within a team are flowing smoothly, quality of life for all involved can skyrocket. You'll never be able to rid your practice of all traces of negativity since they are part of the complicated mixture of the way people naturally are, but the less there is, the better. I am happy to say that my practice currently seems to have an all-time low of these friction points, and I believe that accounts for the quality of life and productivity that we are currently enjoying. It hasn't always been like that, and as I said, it didn't happen by accident.

The word "team" evokes thoughts of sports. Many winning sports coaches will tell you that it is most important to pick a good overall athlete with a winning attitude and a broad range of skills. I believe in that as well. When choosing a new employee, I look for cleanliness, friendliness, character, intelligence, presence, and communication skills. Everything else, I can teach. I "discovered" most of the dental assistants that I've hired working as waitresses. They had impressed me with their ability to present themselves well and interact pleasantly with strangers. All I had to do was teach them what I needed them to do in the office and provide them with the opportunity for further professional training. I consider myself a great teacher in that regard, and in many cases, I was very fortunate in that there was overlap when a new assistant was hired compared to when her predecessor left. That allowed for an effective transfer of information from outgoing to incoming and lessened the transitional downtime. That speaks to the good terms on which most of the people in my employ left when it was time for them to move on.

One of the most overlooked and vital concerns of any business is the cost of acquiring and training new employees. Understanding that should not totally preclude you from terminating when necessary, but it does underscore the need to be extraordinarily careful when selecting a new employee so as to avoid the costly turnover if you choose poorly. There is the cost of the advertising and administrative time setting up the search efforts. There is the sizable cost of diverting the energy and time of you and your employees to train the new person. Most costly of all is the inevitable drop in production you will suffer while either being shorthanded or while waiting for the new person to get up to speed as they learn their way around.

Given that the interpersonal tone of the office has generally been quite good and I think I've been pretty patient during the learning curve, the training process for me has generally been relatively painless. Some were initially much better students and quick learners coming in and were able to process new information in classic ways. Some were passionately competitive and voracious about learning their skills and proving themselves. And finally, there were some whose study skills had never really been fully developed and therefore hid wonderful minds that seemed to grow more and more incredibly capable and impressive with each passing month as their skills improved and their confidence soared. It is also a reflection of the training and communication skills of the outgoing assistants. Most of those outgoing assistants became dental hygienists or full-time college students and left on the very best of terms and in many cases came back to work in my office. I have been fortunate to have had these young women be so helpful in minimizing the hardships of the transitions.

I am proud to have had a hand in the progression of the professional lives of many of these young women who've been involved with my practice over the years. The mentoring and impact upon their lives has been tremendously rewarding to me. I've proudly watched several of them gain citizenship, start families, continue their educations, and achieve financial stability during and after their tenure with me.

After the Love Is Gone

IT'S BEEN said that one bad apple can spoil the bunch. This can certainly happen when it comes to co-worker dynamics. When one person is irrevocably disgruntled, they can pull down the morale of the entire office. Sometimes they do so by pointing out and exaggerating perceived offenses and injustices against themselves and others in the practice in an attempt to garner justification and support for their own side of their conflict. These offenses might be blamed on another employee, resulting in side-taking and division within the organization. Or they may be directed against the owner/boss/dentist. That sort of crusade can be even worse, resulting in contagious mutinous behavior. Leaders should keep an eye open for such negative energy and correct it as quickly as possible. Corrections should be made expeditiously, snuffing out the spark before it burns the whole place down. Correction can mean anything, from something as simple as a conversation all the way up to termination. Ignoring it will eat away at the practice and the quality of life for all involved.

It has been said that in business, one should hire slowly and fire quickly. This is very sage advice. Hiring slowly means hiring carefully with all the proper due diligence. Doing so will hopefully help to reduce problems down the line and render the firing part unnecessary if you've chosen wisely in the beginning. If, however, we make a mistake and a bad one slips in, procrastination in rectifying it will only result in future escalating damage. Splinters can eventually turn to gangrene. I once hired an office manager in an act of desperation without following up on any of her references. Within a week or two, some of her mannerisms, attitudes, and suggestions made me wonder if she was the sort of person I really wanted to be associated with my practice. Although she seemed great during the interview process, once on the job, her attitude toward others was combative and disrespectful. Some of the insurance and billing practices she had employed at other offices were downright fraudulent. After she went home at the end of her first week, I called one of the dentists she had listed as a reference that I was acquainted with but too lazy to call in the first place. I explained my situation, and when I told the doctor the name of the employee, the doctor adamantly insisted that I fire her. I thanked her and told her I would do it first thing Monday. She said, "NO! Do it now! That person is a felon with several aliases, a terrible person who will destroy your practice and its reputation. She is a cancer that needs to be removed immediately." I thanked her for her wise advice and called the employee and told her we were not a good fit and it was not going to work out.

The "hiring slowly and carefully" part is obvious and needs no further explanation. But the firing quickly part is the one that seems to need to be taught. Over the years, it is an inevitable fact that people come and go. I can confidently say that the terminations that came quickly turned out much better and left behind much less residual damage than those that I let drag out. If you have practiced for many years, you have had to fire several employees. It is inevitable. Firing people is never fun. Well, almost never. It's best, when possible, to do it professionally with as little emotion as possible, but to some extent, it is usually somewhat confrontational and rather stressful. I must say, however, that in most cases, especially when the firing is overdue, there is a great sense of relief once it's over. In the long run, it's probably better for all parties involved. You can go about rebuilding without the toxicity and inefficiency. They can, hopefully, find a place they are better suited to, and the rest of the staff can return to a less stressful and more productive environment.

A Fish Rots from the Head First

A MAJOR aspect of setting the tone of the office is leadership. A code of conduct gets established by those in charge. There is an old-world saying that a fish rots from the head first. The rest of the body follows by example. We as the doctor, owner, and leader of the practice dictate the character and standards of our offices. A friendly receptionist and a gentle hygienist are essential, but it is those of us whose name is on the door that truly set the identity of the practice. The way we treat our patients and each other shows others what is expected. And when that type of behavior results in something favorable, it becomes something others will be drawn to and aspire to emulate. We all have our good days and our bad days, but a core of mutual personal and professional respect is essential if a group of people with different personalities and skill sets are to function effectively as a team in such potentially stressful confines like a dental office.

Employees are not the only ones that we need to keep an eye on when it comes to attitude contamination. Practices whose staff seem to be angry and have a lack of empathy for patients, and a void in consideration for each other very often prove to have narcissistic, arrogant, selfish, non-empathetic owners lacking compassion for those around them. Our practices are a reflection of us.

Beyond our practices being a reflection of us, I would like to talk a little about responsibility. These days, everyone in any position of authority claims to take "full responsibility" for their actions or the actions of those under their authority, direction, or command. But what does that actually mean? Do generals or presidents offer to go to prison when someone is inappropriately killed by someone in their command? Do CEOs personally reimburse shareholders fully when they or the people in their organization make errors that cause millions in losses? Of course they don't. But I feel that we as health care providers seem to owe our patients a bit more. Perhaps not an eye for an eye or a tooth for a tooth. But we certainly owe them, for reasons of basic humanity and personal self-respect, our very best efforts to provide them with the best care possible. And when we fall short of achieving that, don't we owe them more than a "not my fault" while looking for the quickest, cheapest, easiest way out of the harsh spotlight of peer review and malpractice court?

We most certainly do. Whether it comes from self-respect, morality, or a competitive attitude to measure up and surpass what is considered average, we should all strive to provide the best care possible, not the bare minimum that we can get away with.

Some of the things that constitute "more than the bare minimum" might include evening follow-up calls, after-hours visits, and various other slightly "over the call of duty" gestures and acts of consideration. As the phrase "a friend in need is a friend indeed" implies, these gestures are most powerful when things aren't going so well for our patients. That is the time to step up and shine, not to shrink away.

The Secret to Success

THROUGHOUT my adult life, I have looked at successful people and tried to figure out what it was that made the difference for them. I have it narrowed down to three simple rules: Don't be a liar. Don't be a jerk. Show up for work. That's it. Now, no one is perfect. We all occasionally approach these lines to some extent. But the less frequently that you do, the easier it is for people to like you and for you to advance in whatever line of work you're in.

"Don't be a liar" is the most clear-cut of the rules. If you lie, you can't be trusted, your word is worth nothing, and over time, your negative reputation will grow and you will eventually become an outcast, unworthy of anyone's respect.

"Don't be a jerk" is much more debatable. There are so many definitions of jerks and so many different situations where different levels of assertiveness versus consideration might be called for. For example, being firm or brusque or even borderline rude, depending on the reason, with a lab or a specialist on behalf of your patient is occasionally appropriate and in fact called for. How firm, how brusque is a matter of situation and opinion. But on the whole, it generally makes more sense to be nice.

"Show up for work" is the most quantifiable of the three. It speaks to opportunity. If you are fortunate enough to have a chance to thrive, you must seize it. You can't turn down the chance to grow your practice and improve your standing in the dental community and community at large. You should take advantage of every chance you get to impress your patients, staff, and colleagues and maintain the forward momentum of your business and professional development. To do so is a measure of your work ethic, strength, vitality, and reliability. You will wear it like a gleaming suit of armor, and people will be inspired and drawn to it whether they realize it or not.

Another way to look at those three categories would be to rephrase them as "be smart or be likeable, or work hard." When you look at many moderately and significantly successful people, they seem to have some favorable blend of high grades in those three categories. Sometimes the grades are balanced. Sometimes they aren't.

Don't get caught up in the math. It's simply a crude method to quantify an explanation of a phenomenon. If you think of a reasonably successful person you know and play with your own grading numbers a bit, I'll bet they come in with a combined slightly above-average grade. Higher combined scores will likely reflect higher levels of success, and they quite likely scored above average in several of the categories. Because if they score above-average in a category, by definition, they are somewhat smarter, more likeable, or harder working than their peers. If they're a little short in one category, and their total was still above-average, they must have made it up in another. If they're incredible in a category, they can probably afford to be weak in another or even both. That's all it takes to win in today's society.

How to Make Them Love You

I'VE THROWN out quite a few anecdotes and thoughts thus far. These are the things that have shaped the person that I've become at the office. I've seen some of the things that worked for me and some of the things that didn't. Quite a few were learned firsthand, while others were shared with me by colleagues or learned at seminars. But most of them were just life skills applied to patient interactions. This following section will outline some of the thought processes I've developed on my pompous, self-aggrandizing journey to popularity and prosperity. I would also say to the dental professionals that read this that I am not trying to dictate what is right or wrong for them to do but rather share some of my observations and opinions. Please do with them as you will.

I know I already covered this ad nauseum, but the value of communication cannot be overstated. It is crucial to speak the specific language of the person you are trying to communicate with. We all know that there is usually more than one acceptable approach to the dental treatment plans we can recommend. Endodontic treatment and crown lengthening versus extractions. Fixed bridgework versus implants. Fillings versus onlays versus crowns, etc. These can be complex decisions dependent on our professional judgments and opinions as well as many other factors. What I'm saying is that what is the best treatment plan for one patient may not be best for another when you consider all of the variables. In addition to the obvious evaluation of the teeth, you must assess the patient as a person. Be realistic about what sort of treatment a medically compromised patient can sit through and endure. Find the most bulletproof solution for the person you have identified as a no-nonsense, definitive person. Consider a more affordable solution for the person who says or hints that they cannot or will not spend a large amount of money. Tailor and sequence your recommendations so that a phobic patient can wrap their head around and face a course of treatment rather than fearfully retreating back home and totally neglecting their dental health even further. Figuring out which of these pathways to choose comes back to our old friend, listening. And assessing. Try to understand what it looks like from their point of view, why they see things the way they do. Maybe you can educate and alter their vision. Many times, unfortunately, you cannot. In those situations, you need to try to do the best you can within the confines of their world.

Sometimes you will have to let an ostrich continue to stick their head in the sand and ignore their problems. In that situation, you will need to use your professional as well as personal and logical judgment so as to determine how truly urgent the recommended dental treatment is. Are we talking about a facial swelling that might close off their airway or the crowning of a "structurally compromised" tooth with a large amalgam restoration in it that could fracture at any time despite having been trouble free for the last fifty years since the filling was placed?

Once you have decided what it is that you recommend to the patient, you must be sufficiently thorough in your explanation. Explain the alternatives, because it is your legal obligation to do so and also to show off the intellectual efforts you have put in on their behalf. Don't forget to include the possible pitfalls. Remember, it's referred to as an explanation to have that conversation beforehand. The exact same conversation conducted after a problem occurs is called an excuse.

Ultimately, it is the patient's final decision as to what to do, and our role is to advise as best as we can.

I think my ability to read people and understand their message started when I was a kid. My elderly grandfather spoke very broken English, and I spoke virtually no Italian, his native language. I would have to pick out the few words I understood, like "tomato plant" or "fig tree," and intently read his face, body language, and tone to fill in the gaps to determine whether he was proud of how they were growing or disappointed with the climate or angry with garden pests like wasps, slugs, or squirrels.

If you're good enough at reading people, you can bridge a gap and get away with saying things other people couldn't. That level of "verbal intimacy" conveys a confidence in the relationship you have established. To do so absolutely demands that you have properly gauged the strength of that relationship and the amount of trust they have in you. You are also showcasing your confidence in their perceived belief of your good intent. It's a gamble, but if you get away with it, it strengthens the relationship and puts the things you say and the treatment you suggest on a higher, more unassailable level. I once stated, without room for discussion, to a dear seventy-eight-year-old patient that he was absolutely getting implants to help stabilize his denture and improve his quality of life. He asked, "Don't I have a choice?" I responded, "Yes, you have a choice. You can either get up and walk next door to the oral surgeon's office or I can hit you over the head and drag you there. That is your choice." As an aside, he walked there, got the implants, and never had a problem with the denture again.

I once told a beautiful woman that her braided hair looked like snakes. And I lived to tell about it. The thing was, she was very nervous and we needed an icebreaker as I walked into the room. My exact words were, "You got that Medusa thing going on." She flashed a shocked glare. I paused, cocked my head, smiled slyly, and then said, "And I like it!" She looked at me, thought about it for a moment, and then giggled, and the panic was shattered. Innately, she knew that I meant it as a compliment and that my fullest intent was to redirect her fearful train of thought and make her feel comfortable.

You would be hard-pressed to find any patients who loved their dentist more than these two. The bottom line is that it's not what you say but how you say it and why.

As to how to make your staff love you, treat them with kindness. Love them, appreciate them, and respect them. Show that they matter and they will run through brick walls and dive in front of bullets for you. Do the opposite and they will put you in front of a brick wall and shoot bullets into you.

Take Charge

SO, WHAT DO you do with all the lessons learned over the years or shared on these pages? And let me reiterate that I've already credited many of the lessons learned to the dentists we worked with, seminar speakers we listened to, and to business advisors and life experiences outside of dentistry. I make very little claim to these as my original thoughts; they are just my personal compilation, interpretation, organization, and application of them. What is it that we can pragmatically do with these ideas to make our practices and our lives more profitable and enjoyable? Finding the answer to that question is the reason I started writing this book. Ultimately, I do think that, in the long run, we can have a strong influence on our odds for success and happiness. In fact, I am fully confident that I can further influence my world as I continue to practice by taking heed of the lessons learned. A more pessimistic person would be quick to lament the fact that it took so long to learn these things. "If I only knew then what I know now," they would complain. Understand that you cannot change the past. You can only learn from your experiences and lessons and use them to impact and, hopefully, improve your future.

One such observation that occurred was at a dinner meeting many years ago. There were about eight dentists sitting around the table. There was one loudmouthed, sloppily dressed, boorish slob of a dentist monopolizing the conversation. He was bragging about how many specialty procedures he was skilled enough to do himself without giving away the patients and the money to endodontists, periodontists, and oral surgeons. He also stated as fact that anyone who spent more than thirty minutes for a crown prep appointment was slow and foolish. He spent the other half of his self-appointed unlimited speaking time complaining about his patients. He whined that they complained about how he hurt them and about how his crowns looked and felt. He even had the cluelessness to grumble about the fact that his patients complained about his crowns falling out. The ironically hilarious part of it all was that, with every word that he spoke in an effort to set himself above his peers, he inadvertently painted an uglier and uglier pathetic portrait of himself and the quality of his work and the relationship he had with his patients. There was a stink of negativity to him, and his bragging was a vain attempt to hide his unhappiness. He clearly hated his patients, and many of them undoubtedly hated him too. He seemed easy to dislike.

By comparison, there was a well-dressed older dentist at the table. He was probably in his late sixties, and he had a soft-spoken, classy, professional demeanor. When interrogated by the slob about how long he took for a crown appointment, he said ninety minutes. When the slob laughed at him and pressed him to join into his vitriolic diatribe about his patients, he simply replied that his patients were his friends and he was fortunate to have them.

So, by whatever means it took, this dentist seemed to have cultivated a much more pleasant environment for himself and his staff. Perhaps he did it by setting a code of behavior that his staff and patients followed. Maybe he somehow found a way to dismiss or not attract so many negative patients. Most likely, he was just a man of high character and carried that into most aspects of his life. I'm not sure, but the one thing that I was certain of from that day on was that his was the type of practice I would seek to emulate, not the slob's.

I feel it is imperative to obtain a clear and honest vision of your practice, your life, and yourself. Use that vision as an accurate starting point and assessment of what can truly be achieved. You have a lot more control in the attainment of that than you think you have. I've talked about how to visualize and build the practice you want, but now let's talk about how to maintain and improve it. For starters, recognize and pull the weeds. No garden is productive and no lawn is beautiful when cluttered with energy-sucking, poisonous weeds. It is much better in the long run to pull them out, even if you have to get your hands dirty and leave a bit of a bare spot for a little while. It will grow back in much healthier than before.

Become a strong judge of character and human nature, and apply that knowledge as a predictor of how someone will continue to behave. Be critical of facts and statements told to you. Lying is an ugly word. Exaggerating, bluffing, omitting the truth, and deflectors of blame all come from much less evil branches of the same family tree, and all can lead to problems if you completely believe them. Many times, the person saying these things does not see the intrinsic dishonesty in the things they are saying. In fact, they often believe it themselves.

You don't need to shun all people who engage in any of these deviations from the absolute truth, but you do need to recognize and keep in perspective facts and statements that may be a little less than 100 percent truthful. A perfect example is someone who tells you to bet on a certain racehorse, saying things like "It's a lock!" "Guaranteed!" Should you really empty out your bank account and bet everything you own on that horse? Is it so "guaranteed" that he will reimburse your losses if the horse doesn't win? I doubt it.

Similarly, when a patient with a lifetime of neglect of their teeth and most other affairs of their life comes to your office and declares that they suddenly want to fully restore all of their teeth for tens of thousands of dollars, should you cancel all of your other patients for the next few weeks and place an order for a new luxury car? Probably not. It is neither a lock nor is it guaranteed. In fact, experience will teach you that it's rather unlikely. I'm not saying you should call them a liar and chase them out of your office; just be realistic as to the validity of their statements and the impact you let them exert on your life. With regard to staff members and specialists that you work with, a zero-tolerance policy for lying should be followed due to the direct impact it has on the quality of the care you are able to provide to the patient.

"Control Your Implant Cases or They Will Control You"

LARGE RESTORATIVE implant cases can really test your abilities regarding the concepts of controlling your world and visualizing the true intent of patients. The stakes are high. These cases can be lengthy, expensive, and complicated. They can be frightening to our patients and demand advanced communication and clinical skills to navigate successfully. And by "successfully," I mean several things. First and foremost, it means that you can provide a solid restoration that enhances the life of your patient. But it also means that you can do it in a fashion that does not endlessly torture or bankrupt you or your patient unnecessarily. Lack of expertise or poor planning and communication can easily cause disaster. Perhaps the most important thing I ever heard a seminar speaker say was "Control your implant cases, or they will control you." Brilliant and true. The same implant case that, when properly handled, simply involves assembly and insertion of precise components, like building a Lego toy, can turn into a nightmare of endless appointments, apologies, and astronomical lab and component expenses when not properly controlled. And the worst part of some of these nightmare cases is that there is virtually no chance of success at the end of it. And you realize this fact halfway through this costly, poorly planned journey.

The very first step of this control starts when evaluating the case to determine the very feasibility of it. Be sure to recognize and consider all potential threats to its success and be very pragmatic and honest with yourself when you assess the likelihood and severity of them. Lack of adequate bone where you need it or implants carelessly or improperly placed that cannot sufficiently support your intended restoration can doom you before you begin. The concept of restorative-driven placement was a godsend to us restorative dentists, and we are foolish if we do not embrace it, live by it, and demand it from our surgeons. It demands focus, concentration, and performance from our surgical colleagues, with a clear understanding and vision of the final restoration. Too many times, we have implants sent to us in the wrong place, and we are asked to make it work. All too often, we are tempted to try to be a hero and try to make it work against all odds. There's a good reason for odds, and let's not forget that no good deed goes unpunished. There is no Good Samaritan law in effect here. Once things fail, everyone shares the blame, regardless of who caused it.

The next critical step is to properly convey all of the aspects of the projected treatment to your patient. Do not sugarcoat or omit details. Best to discuss unpleasantries like possible additional costs or failed implants while they are still explanations rather than excuses. Between the wasted chair time and the additional costs you would otherwise be compelled to absorb, believe me when I say that the timing of these discussions will save you a ton of money and shame. And yes, in case I haven't mentioned it enough times yet, communication is key. Not only to tell your patient everything you need to tell them but also to completely hear and gauge their commitment of time, effort, and money to the completion of treatment. This is not a battle for deserters, so make sure you see the commitment in their eyes.

How to Grow

THE CONCEPT of how to grow a practice can be argued and debated endlessly. The only fact that all parties would agree upon is that dental practices are like any other businesses in that they need to acquire new patients to replace those that they lose. Some level of loss is inevitable. Patients move away, they die, they choose another dentist. It's life. It happens. Most would also agree that it is just as important to retain the patients you already have so as to lessen the need to acquire new ones. How to get new ones is truly a matter of opinion, and I am not here to call anyone wrong. What is also a matter of opinion is whether long-term retention of patients whose dentistry has all been done is more or less valuable than the acquisition of new patients with more work to be done. A lot could be discussed on both sides of that issue.

As to the various methods of marketing and the acquisition of new patients, what has always served me well is internal marketing and word of mouth. While that may sound old-fashioned, homespun, and cheap, it works. Not necessarily for hordes of new patients per month but certainly for a more stable long-term solution. Keeping your existing patient base happy, feeling appreciated, and enthusiastic not only promotes stability and cash flow but also encourages them to refer friends and family. These new people come in with a two-step head start into the relationship building. They have already been told good things about me from someone whose opinion they trust, and I can be pretty confident that a good patient of mine would not send someone they know to be a nightmare to my office. In fact, most people tend to associate with and listen to the recommendations of people like themselves. It's been my experience that good people refer good people and bad refer bad.

If this method does not seem to generate an adequate new patient flow on its own, additional measures can be taken to boost it a bit. Recognizing who seems to be an enthusiastic advocate of your practice and encouraging future referrals from them is always a good idea. These people are referred to as mavens, and the relationships with these people are incredibly valuable to the internal, grassroots growth of a practice. It's also been said that, if you want more patients, just ask for them. When a patient tells you how much they love you or your office, thank them, and tell them to refer a friend. Ask why their husband doesn't come here or why their eighteen-year-old kid still goes to the pedodontist.

Friends and relatives are very much a mixed bag as patients. It's very nice to take care of them, and there is usually enough profitability to do so, but in the big picture, it's not always a good idea to do business with friends. It can be awkward if things don't go as perfectly as everyone would like, but on the other hand, they can and will be your most enthusiastic referral sources. This call is truly debatable, and I can't say I have a definitive opinion either way. You should consider the pros and cons and decide which applies to you.

While internal marketing is indeed my personal favorite and is responsible for more of our new patients, you absolutely need a multifaceted approach to growth efforts. It's simply too important to put all your eggs in one basket, and you only have just so many existing patients able to sing your praises. This is why you cannot count on a continued source of new patients from word of mouth heavy enough to balance the attrition as well as fuel new growth. In this day and age, it is essential to have some online presence, as today's consumers always look to the internet for a broader, more convenient view of the services they need.

Expanded hours were quite the rage before Covid. I think their importance waned a little once people were working from home and a little more available during the week. I suppose some of that will revert. Expanded hours do come with a bit of good news and bad news. The good news is that, if your office is open nights and weekends, you are more likely to attract those who could not or would not come during traditional business hours. One could argue that, for certain procedures like emergency care or major restorative and surgical care, patients will make the time to come in during the day. But preventative care, like cleanings for the entire family, certainly thrives on Saturdays. And evening appointments for working people on their way home from work are always popular. As a dentist/owner, you have to weigh the importance of a strong preventative practice against the loss of your social leisure time and try to find the balance between the two that suits you best. When doing these calculations, one must also consider the low popularity of having to work these times among staff. Another problem with Saturdays is that some people book these times long in advance because they don't place a very high priority on it and figure they won't have anything better to do that day. Once the day draws near and their social calendar starts to fill up or the weather looks nice and they have something better to do that day, they bail, and you find yourself wondering why you gave up your day off.

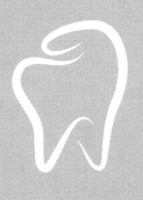

PART THREE

IN CONCLUSION

Mind Control

WE SOMETIMES find ourselves struggling to find a way to make it through a difficult day or some seemingly overwhelming task. Sometimes we feel stalemated as we attempt to wrap our head around the entirety of a complex case or challenge. At times, it is best to look outside our instinctive comprehensive mindset in situations like these. You see, we are trained to be worriers, micromanagers who agonize over every detail and constantly evaluate the odds for success. We are control freaks. In fact, I've already told you to do these things several times in this very book. But sometimes, we need to step away from that sort of thinking. We need to think like a Navy SEAL and focus on and accomplish each task, one at a time, aiming directly at the one at hand without worrying about and becoming paralyzed by things in the distant future. We need to devour that elephant the only way a person can. One bite at a time. Being distracted or intimidated by the size or scope of the project or things that haven't even happened yet and may not happen can derail you and prevent you from completing the very manageable current assignment. And while you are focusing on the task at hand, do it right. Greatness is not about doing one amazing thing one time. It's about doing one hundred small things one percent better one hundred times.

At the end of the day, this business is about people. For people, by people, with people, and despite people. The human element with all of its extremes is omnipresent in what we do. We deal with it much more so than many other professions. Confidence, fear, compassion, logic, leadership, and a host of others are all in there. The dynamics and interactions can be overwhelming. You must manage these traits in yourself and those around you or at least recognize, understand, and cope with them. Being the ringmaster in this circus can often feel like emotional dodgeball. You have to cheerfully withstand this barrage of concerns and find a solution and take care of everyone. It's why we go home tired at the end of the day. It's why bosses get paid more money. But is it enough? Is it worth it? In the long run, it probably isn't. That is a philosophical discussion for another book. That's why it's best to try to eliminate or at least minimize the stressors rather than just nickel-and-diming your way up a few dollars to try to make that pummeling a little more survivable.

Once the toxicity is at least diminished in your life and you can look ahead with a clear optimistic vision, I believe a combination of two components is essential. One is passion, and the other is pragmatism. If you are passionate about what you do, your enthusiasm will rise. Productivity will remain high, and prosperity will follow. You will be happy, and as they say, "If you love what you do, you will never work a day in your life." That said, a certain amount of pragmatism needs to be blended into the mix. Let's be adults about this. You can't trade the family cow for a handful of magic beans. Different dentists bring a different blend of these two essential elements to the mix, but you certainly need some of both in order to do what we do for a living.

I believe that it starts with the type of person you inherently are. You can modify and cultivate certain traits, but at your core, you are who you are. Too much of an attempt to be someone you aren't will be transparent and unimpressive. Confidence is a trait that is essential in most of what we do. It is more than brashness or watered-down arrogance. It is more about believing in yourself and what you do. Knowing that you will keep your word makes your promises more believable. Unless you are an incredible liar, there is nothing quite so unquestionable as the truth. Knowing deep in your core that you will do the very best you can shows through when you speak to a patient and encourage them to follow your recommendations. In fact, on some level, I appreciate having to redo some of my own work occasionally when I feel it does not live up to my standards. The taste of that redo powerfully fortifies my sincerity when I tell the next patient that I stand unconditionally behind my work and my promises. Patients can sense that sincerity and are therefore more inclined to follow your recommendations.

Once you solidify your self-esteem and hold yourself to a higher standard, your standing in the dental community as well as the general community will be elevated. You will enjoy more positive experiences in other aspects and interactions in your life. Your good reputation will become a self-fulfilling prophecy. It may manifest itself quantifiably as more patient referrals to your office or as something more intangible (but every bit as important) as people telling your five-year-old daughter what a wonderful dentist her dad is. A great reputation like that takes quite a while to establish. A bad reputation, on the other hand, can happen very quickly and can ruin a practice and crush your self-esteem. So do the right thing for your patients, and don't let subpar work and misdeeds walk around town with your name on it.

You want to leave a legacy and have those closest to you be proud of you. It enhances their lives as well as yours. At one point, while I was in dental school and contemplating quitting, one of my uncles called me "Doc" with such a prideful grin that I instantly knew quitting was not an option. I didn't quit, and things worked out quite well for me. The point is that obligations, pride, and reinforcement from those around us all go hand in hand. You're not in this alone, and it's not all about you. A strong, honest self-awareness and an understanding as to how you fit into society are truly powerful things.

Two-Minute Warning

SO HERE we are. Thirty-eight years in, and a few to go. What have I learned? What comes next, and how can I affect the outcome? There's a joke that goes, "How do you know you are at a ridiculous cockfight? The answer is "there's a duck entered." Wait for the mild chuckle . . . "How do you know crooks are involved?" "The duck wins."

I'm not a crook, but I like it when the duck wins. I like predictability and increasing my odds of a positive outcome. I like a rigged game where the odds are in my favor and a win is almost certain. I believe that following a lot of the principles outlined in this book can help to tilt the odds a bit in your favor—kind of like counting cards in blackjack.

So how do I make the very best of the last years of practice and not leave things up to chance? Not quite ready to leave our practices and the role that has defined us for several decades, many of my colleagues and I at this stage of the game might like to practice a bit longer but would also like to enjoy it more. Perhaps we feel we have earned that right. And possibly, we would like to think that a lesson or two has gotten through our thick heads and enabled us to do what we do a bit more efficiently and with a little less frustration. There are certainly a few more people we feel uniquely capable of helping and possibly a few more heartwarming and amusing stories to be gathered.

So, I ask one last time. What is the purpose of this book? Is it a road map for the rest of my time practicing? Or maybe it's a "How-to" book for young dentists? Sort of a "If I knew then what I know now" thing. I think it would be helpful to a younger generation of dentists early in their careers, but old people always say that. There was nothing truly earth-shattering in here. No divine revelations or magic formulas. But life is never about magic formulas. It's about applying things you've learned in the past to situations you find yourself in now.

There was no story told here so unique that most experienced dentists could not relate to or top. I would like to think it was a bit insightful and occasionally somewhat entertaining. Maybe it was just a walk down memory lane. Or perhaps it's a glance at the scoreboard and the wrinkled, coffee-stained playbook late in the game as I ask myself what I've accomplished. And how I can finish strong with my head held high.

Thanks for reading.

Made in the USA
Middletown, DE
01 August 2024

58333611R00082